MAXILLOFACIAL SURGERY

Edited by **Leon A. Assael**

Maxillofacial Surgery
http://dx.doi.org/10.5772/1650
Edited by Leon Assael

Contributors

Maria Piagkou, Theano Demesticha, Giannoulis Piagkos, Panayiotis Skandalakis, Elizabeth Johnson, Babatunde Akinbami, Everton Da Rosa, Júlio Evangelista De Souza Júnior, Melina Spinosa Tiussi, Raphael R. Ciuman, Philipp Dost

First published in Croatia, 2012 by INTECH d.o.o.
eBook (PDF) Published by IN TECH d.o.o.
Place and year of publication of eBook (PDF): Rijeka, 2019.
IntechOpen is the global imprint of IN TECH d.o.o.
Printed in Croatia

Legal deposit, Croatia: National and University Library in Zagreb

Additional hard and PDF copies can be obtained from orders@intechopen.com

Maxillofacial Surgery
Edited by Leon Assael

p. cm.

ISBN 978-953-51-0627-2

eBook (PDF) ISBN 978-953-51-7002-0

Meet the editor

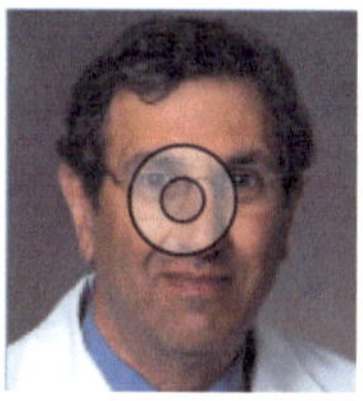

Dr Leon A. Assael AB, DMD, FACD, FICD is Professor and Chairman of Oral and Maxillofacial Surgery, Residency Program Director, and Medical Director Hospital Dentistry and Professor of Surgery OHSU Schools of Medicine and Dentistry in Portland, Oregon. Dr Assael is an alumnus of Columbia University (AB in government), Harvard University (DMD), Vanderbilt University (residency in OMS) and the University of Kentucky (CMM). He is certified by the American Board of Oral and Maxillofacial Surgery. He served as Dean of the University Of Kentucky College Of Dentistry from 1997-2003. He was also on the faculty of the University of Connecticut from 1989-1997 and served as department head in surgical sciences and Associate Chief of Staff of the John Dempsey Hospital. From 1981-1989, he was residency program director in oral and maxillofacial surgery at the Mount Sinai School of Medicine. Dr Assael is the past Editor in Chief of the Journal of Oral and Maxillofacial Surgery. He is the past Chairman of the Council on Dental Education and Licensure of the American Dental Association. He is the recipient of several national and international awards including The Donald Osbon award for outstanding educator, the William F. Harrigan award, and the Kurt Thoma award. He has also delivered lectureships honoring leaders in oral and maxillofacial surgery including William Ware, Sadie Fontaine, Peter Connole, Ben Alley, and Daniel Waite. In 2001, President George W. Bush awarded Dr Assael the America's Promise award for advancements in oral health in Appalachia achieved by the faculty of the University of Kentucky. In 2010, the American Association of Oral and Maxillofacial Surgeons awarded Dr Assael the Board of Trustees special recognition award. The author of textbooks including books on temporomandibular disorders, cleft lip and palate and facial injuries, and over 100 peer reviewed contributions to the scientific literature.

Contents

Preface

Oral and maxillofacial surgery is a specialty rooted in dentistry and forged in academic medical centers in departments of surgery, as the surgical specialty well equipped to care for conditions of the mouth, jaws, head and neck. Today oral and maxillofacial surgeons are advancing cancer care, neurosciences, understanding the pathology of the region, managing congenital and acquired deformities among others. In the process this specialty is improving the lives of our patients with better function, appearance, self esteem and longevity.

This text is unique in that it is developed online and published in that fashion. It also addresses some unique issues that are important subsets of the needs of oral and maxillofacial surgery patients. While it does not comprehensively address the field, the papers enclosed provide an important niche in the development of the future specialty of oral and maxillofacial surgery

Dr. Leon A. Assael
Oregon Health and Science University,
USA

1

Radiologic Evaluation, Principles of Management, Treatment Modalities and Complications of Orofacial Infections

Babatunde O. Akinbami
Department of Oral and Maxillofacial Surgery,
University of Port Harcourt Teaching Hospital, Rivers State,
Nigeria

1. Introduction

1.1 Radiological evaluation of orofacial infection

- Intraoral x-rays

Periapical view is useful to show the affected tooth/ teeth crown, root apex in cases of caries, fracture, impaction and periodontitis

Occlusal view is useful to show any stone in the submandibular salivary gland which may cause an ascending infection in the gland and later spread to the soft tissue space

- Plain soft tissue x-rays of the skull, jaws and neck are useful to see expansions in the soft tissue spaces in the head and neck region.

Also plain hard tissue x-rays such as the tangential Posterior-anterior view can show calculi in the parotid duct

Conventional posterior-anterior, oblique laterals are useful to show mixed osteolytic changes (radiolucencies) and new bone formation (radioopacities) in chronic osteomyelitis of the mandible; which is the classical moth eaten appearance.

For the maxilla, occipitomental and true lateral views are useful.

However, a single view of orthopantomogram (panorex) is useful for both mandible and maxilla

- Chest x-rays
- Computerized tomographic scan is mainly useful for bone lesions as in osteomyelitis giving reduced CT no. in areas of bone destruction and close to normal CT no. in areas of bone formation. Fluids, abscesses and exudates gives varying opacities and lucencies with CT no. more than that of water (0) and cerebrospinal fluid (7) but less than fat (100) and bone (1000).

1.2 Types of CT scans

1. Traditional or single slice CT scan- produces single slice of images from the data obtained from detectors in the gantry. The patient's table must be turned to allow another 360 degrees revolution for a second slice of 3mm or less to be made.
2. Spiral CT scan- Allows simultaneous movement of table and x-ray tube; has a single row of detectors which produces volumetric data set and allows reconstruction of multiple slices of images obtained in a single revolution. The images can also be reformatted and viewed in multiple planes with the Pictural archival communication system. Also has the advantage of less artifact due to swallowing because a single breathe hold is utilized, gives better vascular opacification and small contrast bolus is needed to enhance lesions.
3. Multi-detector CT scan- has a matrix of detectors which sends volumetric data sets to produce multiple slices of images in more than the three planes at one revolution thereby increasing the speed of imaging.
4. New Tom CT scan (Schick, NIM, S.r.l., Verona, Italy) produces axial panoramic images and 3D data set for multiplanar images. It is a cone-beam CT scan which apart from the 3D dimensional imaging produced, also exposes patients to less radiations, but not useful for inflammatory swellings.
5. Contrast enhanced CT. scan- Contrast is introduced to enhance imaging of soft tissue space infections.

- Magnetic resonance imaging clearly demarcates the exudates accumulation and expansions within the soft tissue compartments. In the T2 weighted sequence image, soft tissue space swellings appear more opaque than the soft tissues while the bones appear dark.

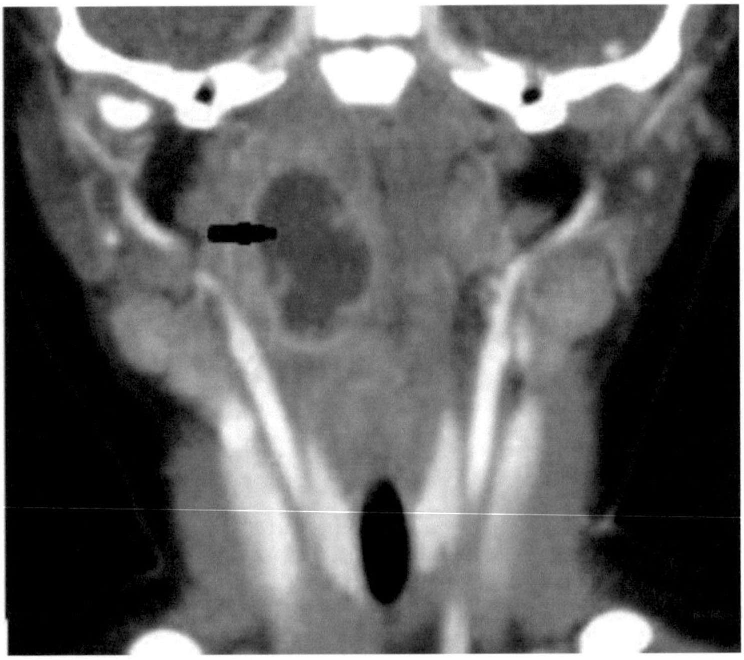

Fig. 1. Shows CT scan demonstrating a retropharygeal abscess; excerpt from anaerobicinfections.blogspot.com

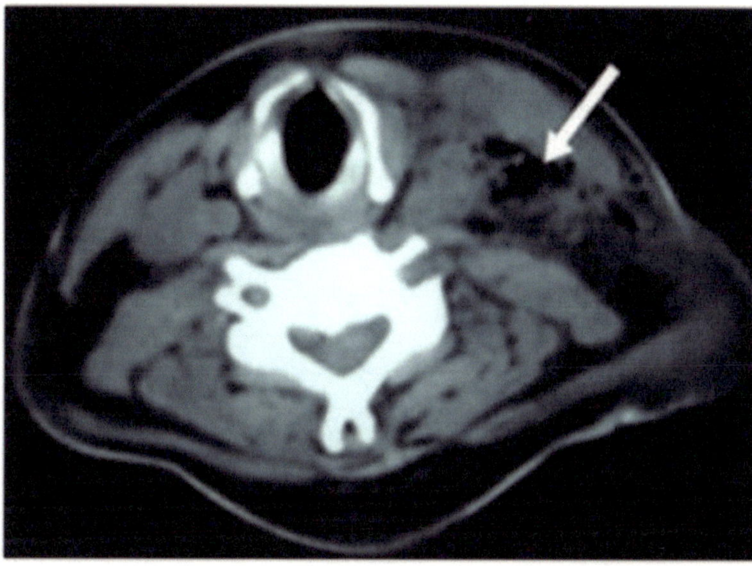

Fig. 2. Shows CT scan demonstrating a collection of gas filled abscess in the neck; excerpt from anaerobicinfections.blogspot.com

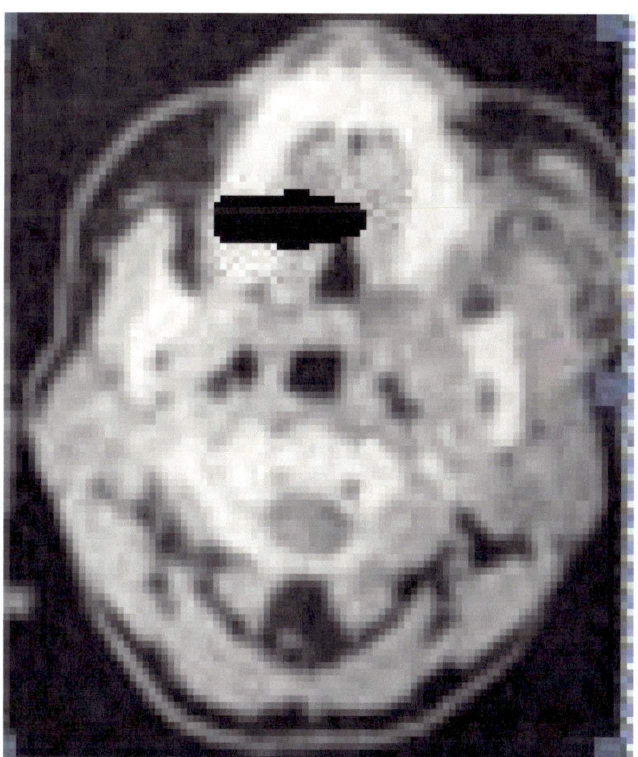

Fig. 3. Shows Contrast enhanced CT scan demonstrating a sublingual space abscess

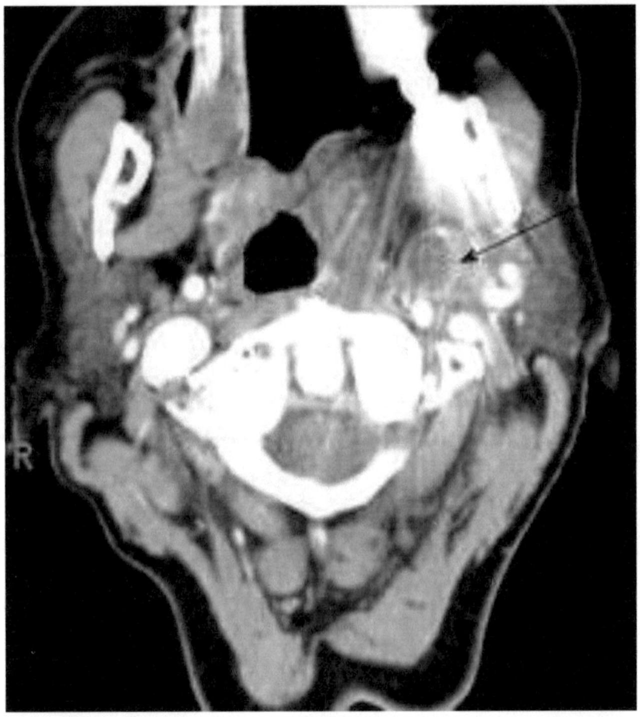

Fig. 4. Shows Contrast enhanced CT scan demonstrating left parapharygeal space abscess excerpt from abcradiology.blogspot.com

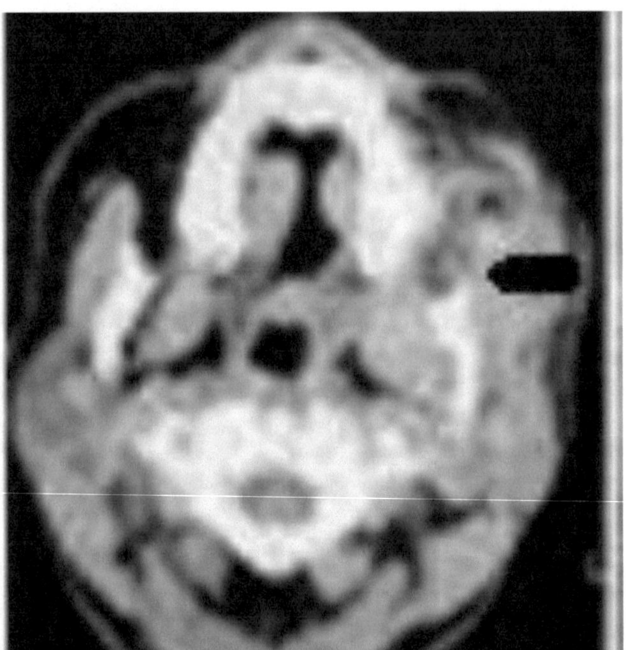

Fig. 5. Shows Contrast enhanced CT scan demonstrating a left buccal space abscess

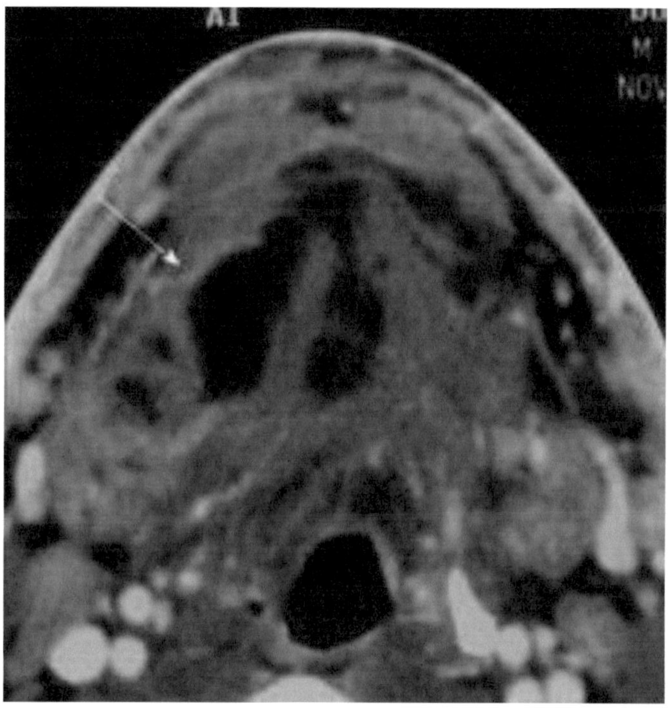

Fig. 6. Shows Contrast enhanced CT scan demonstrating multiple abscess in Ludwig's angina; excerpt from abcradiology.blogspot.com

- Ultrasound scan is also useful for superficial soft tissue imaging with probes of high frequencies of 7.5Mhz and above
- Scintiscanning is very useful to ascertain the presence of exudates within bone especially in the early phase as well as in the established phase of acute osteomyelitis, producing high signals in the spectrum of that of inflammations. X-rays and CT scans may not be very useful in acute osteomyelitis to demonstrate early bone changes.

Soft tissues and exudates are best evaluated using contrast medium, therefore the best imaging technique is contrast CT-scan. The soft tissues, spaces and exudates appear radioopaque on contrast CT scans. Moreover, CT scan is cheaper, readily available and has no electromagnetic effects on patients with metallic implants compared to MRI and most patients do not react to the contrast medium (Gadolinium) which is injected into the body via intravenous route before the scan. Pre-operative and post- operative evaluation of the lesions/swellings by these imaging modalities not only assist in the diagnosis but also serve as a guide in the treatment and monitoring of progress. Incision and decompression, sequestrectomies are now being done under ultrasonic and CT guidance.

2. Principles of treatment and treatment modalities of orofacial infection

Thorough evaluation of the patients with these infections, elimination of local factors and control of systemic diseases contribute to the successful management and good outcome. Effective decompression, choice and dosages of antibiotics, compliance of patients are measures necessary to combat these problems with a view to reducing the morbidity and mortality.

The spread of the infections in patients with periapical periodontitis and dentoalveolar abscess who present early to the hospital is better curtailed with empirical broad spectrum oral antibiotics within five days to 1 week.

- Capsule amoxycillin 500mg or amoxycillin/clavulanate and
- Tablet metronidazole 400mg 8hrly
- Analgesic tablet paracetamol or ibuprufen

For infections that have spread to the potential spaces;

- It is better to admit;
- Commence empirical intravenous antibiotics,

No gold standard for antibiotic regime, based on the polymicrobial etiologic nature of odontogenic infections, patients can be given

- intravenous metronidazole 500mg/100ml 8hrly for 72hrs
- with intravenous broad spectrum antibiotic amoxycillin/clavulanate or ceftriaxone commenced before the outcome of the m/c/s results.

Parenteral Analgesics;

- either paracetamol or
- selective cyclo-oxygenase enzyme inhibitor, non- steroidal anti-inflammatory drugs; celecoxib or
- non-selective, diclofenac with misoprostol to protect the gastric/duodenal wall.

Rehydrate with intravenous fluids, Dextrose saline 5% alternate with Normal saline 0.9% 1 liter 8hrly for 72hrs, fluid control however should be depend on degree of dehydration, renal status, input/output chart. An average output of 1-2mls per minute per kg body weight must be maintained.

3. Principles of drainage

Drain abscesses both intraorally or extraorally depending on the site.

Drainage may be done under conscious sedation or general anaesthesia depending on the extent of spread, airway obstruction, patients' cooperation and availability of facilities and necessary skills

For cases to be done under G.A, orotracheal or fibreoptic intubation without muscle relaxants is preferred to prevent further compromise of the airway. Both forms of intubation can enhance quicker access or visibility into the airway than nasotracheal.

If there is airway obstruction, cricothyrostomy or tracheostomy may be necessary.

3.1 Procedure

1. Make about 1.5 - 2cm skin incision in the most dependent fluctuant site/sites on the swelling to aid drainage under gravity where possible.
2. Blunt dissection into the swelling, the swelling is entered with the sinus forceps closed and then opened and moved in different directions to break multiple loci of pus, drainage is aided with digital pressure, suction and can be guided by radiologic or endoscopic imaging
3. After satisfactory decompression of exudates, sinus forceps should be removed with the beaks wide open to avoid gripping of any vital tissue.

- For submandibular and Ludwig's abscesses, the first layer is skin followed by the subcutaneous tissue and platysma muscle within it, then the outer part of the investing layer of deep cervical fascia before entering into the submandibular space which is below the inner part of the investing layer. Further dissection through the inner part and mylo-hyoid muscle which forms the floor of the mouth allows access into the sublingual space which is below the oral mucosa. Dissections should be along same line and at least 3cm away from the lower border of the mandible to avoid the salivary glands. At least 3 interrupted incisions are made for ludwig's angina.
- For submasseteric abscesses, approach can be transoral (intraoral) or via the neck (extraoral) or both. Extraoral can be retromandibular- this also allow drainage of intermuscular planes easily without going through masseter muscle but continuous drainage is not aided by gravity and extra care must be taken to protect the retromandibular vein, external carotid artery, and facial nerve. The submandibular offers access below the angle of the mandible avoiding those structures and drainage under gravity is better but dissection is through the muscle. Intraoral dissection may be added to facilitate drainage and incision is made on mucosa along the anterior border of the ramus of mandible, sinus forceps is inserted into the space lateral to the ramus and medial to masseter
- For pterygomandibular space, same intraoral incision at same site allows penetration into the space, which is medial to the ramus and lateral to the medial pterygoid.

- For lateral pharyngeal space, same incision, also allow forceps into the space lateral to the superior constrictor and medial to the medial pterygoid.
- For infratemporal space, the incision is extended higher to the coronoid process, the forceps penetrates medial to the attachment of the temporalis muscle and below the lateral pterygoid muscle. Care must be taken to avoid the internal maxillary vessels, mandibular nerve/branches and pterygoid plexus.
- For peritonsillar space abscess (Quinsy), incision is made into the mucosa in the tonsillar bed anterior to the tonsils, quick suctioning of the exudates must be done to avoid aspirations.

By the second day of admission, when the patient is fairly stable,

- Extractions of the causal tooth/teeth should be done and
- Commence jaw exercises with mouth gag to continue daily with wooden spatula- this will improve the mouth opening and aid the drainage of exudate.

By the end of the third day or beginning of fourth day, Empirical antibiotic given needed to be changed after the arrival of the m/c/s result if response is not satisfactory. Patients with spreading soft tissue space infections and bone infections have to be admitted for about two to three weeks.

4. Treatment modalities of osteomyelitis

All cases of suppurative osteomyelitis must be admitted.

Those with acute suppurative osteomyelitis are to commence on fluids and intramuscular analgesics and empirical antibiotics while waiting for M/C/S result.

Intravenous Sparxfloxacin 200mg 12 hrly for 72hrs with lincomycin 500mg 8hrly or clindamycin 300mg 12hrly for 4 weeks. If symptoms of necrotizing colitis start, the macrolides should be stopped.

Those with chronic suppurative osteomyelitis must wait for M/C/S result before given antibiotic-no need for empirical antibiotics

Also indicated for chronic osteomyelitis is

1. sequestrectomy and
2. excision of the sinus tracts.

4.1 Focal sclerosing osteomyelitis

May not need any intervention but if there is persistent pain or superimposed infection,

- Extraction of tooth/teeth
- Excision of sclerotic bone, place autograft or allograft bone material if necessary
- Antibiotic coverage

4.2 Chronic sclerosing osteomyelitis

There have been controversies over the origin and aetiology of diffuse sclerosing osteomyelitis. Some authors believe that it is due to organisms like *propionibacterium acne and peptostreptococcus intermedius* found in the deep pockets associated with generalized periodontitis. Others believe that it may be part of a bone, joint and skin {SAPHO; synovitis, acne, pustulosis, hyperostosis and osteitis} syndrome probably due to allergic or autoimmune reaction in the periosteum[7].

Based on this fact, it has been found that

- Corticosteroids or high doses of potent NSAIDs and biphosphonates have been useful in its management;
- With or without prolonged antibiotic therapy and
- Decortications as well as thorough
- Periodontal tissue management with
- Oral hygiene instructions.

4.3 Refractory osteomyelitis

In refractory cases, not responsive to the above treatment, resection of that part of bone involved and reconstruction with bone grafts with or without alloplastic bone substitutes and reconstruction plates will be indicated

- Occasionally, hyperbaric oxygen daily for 1 month may also be required.

The average period of antibiotic coverage for the patients with soft tissue space infections and dentoalveolar abscess ranged between 5 to 14days while that for osteomyelitis was between 4 to 6 weeks. The latest broad spectrum antibiotics now used in the treatment of orofacial infections are the fourth generation cephalosporins (Cefepime) and the Imipenems/ cilastin derivatives (Bacqure). Both are exceptional in the treatment of beta lactamase producing organisms.

5. Complications of orofacial infections

5.1 Early complications

1. Regional and distant spread (abscess in any part of the body)-

Spread of odontogenic infections accounts for up to 57 % of deep neck abscesses (Mihos et al., 2004). With the potential for infection spreading to the interpleural space and mediastinal tissue, the mortality rate of mediastinitis continues to be 17–50 % despite aggressive use of antibiotics and advances in intensive care facilities (Marty-Ane et al., 1999).

- Additional incisions below the swellings have to be made for patients whose infection had spread to the neck and chest wall, to allow for drainage
- For spread into the thorax, a chest tube will be needed at the seventh intercostal space mid-axillary line or a thoracotomy when there is organisation and consolidation
- Paracentesis/laparatomy for abbominal/pelvic abscesses
- Orbital decompression will be needed for spreading retrobulbar abscess
- Cranial burr holes/craniotomy for intracranial abscess

2. **Septicemia and Toxic shock syndrome**- recognized by high temperature, pallor, jaundice, increasing respiratory and pulse rate with reducing blood pressure. Massive

and aggressive intravenous antibiotics, intravenous fluids and diet (hyperalimentation), hyperbaric oxygen and ozone therapy application may be useful but with the risk of pulmonary toxity.

3. Necrotizing fascitis marked by erythema, blistering and denudation/loss of skin, subcutaneous tissue, deep fascia and muscle due to devitalization- Excision of devitalized tissue and repititive debridemole must be done combined with intravenous antibiotics and antiseptic dressings. High protein diet and fluid intake as well as control of systemic factors are vital. Biotherapy with honey and larvatherapy are also applicable.
4. **Disseminated intravascular coagulopathy** marked by blood coming out from all orifices in the body; Blood, fresh frozen plasma, cryoprecipitate and factor VIII and platelet concentrate must be given.
5. **Cavernose sinus thrombosis** marked by severe headache, vomiting, high temperature, redness, proptosis and painful swelling of the eyeball/lid and prominent conjunctival and schlera vessels- Massive and aggressive intravenous antibiotics with anti-inflammatory analgesics must be given, subcutaneous low dose heparin, intravenous fluids and diet
6. Chronic suppurative otitis media and mastoditis
7. **Stroke (embolic)**- Appropriate consult.
8. **Death -** Death usually occurs due to sepsis and multi-organ failure although airway occlusion is also a significant complication and requires early management by tracheostomy. Host factors affected by the patient's general health condition play a significant role.

5.2 Late complications

1. Ankylosis of the temporomandibular joint
2. Myositis ossificans and
3. Subperiostitis osteomyelitis- the last two is common with improper treated submassetric abscess
4. Bone destruction and facial deformities
5. Blindness and deafness.

In the study of Akinbami et al., hospitalized patients were rehydrated with intravenous fluids, 5% dextrose/saline alternate with 0.9% normal saline 1litre 8hrly for 72 hrs. Dextrose fluid was avoided in patients treated for diabetics. 10 I.U of subcutaneous insulin (humulin) 4hrly was commenced for patients with diabetis mellitus and physicians were consulted to continue management. The mortality figure was 11.8%. In most studies reviewed, caries was the most predominant local factor, while diabetic mellitus and malnutrition were commonest systemic diseases.

6. Conclusion

Control of systemic factors/diseases is a vital and integral component in the management of these patients with orofacial infections, therefore holistic approach must be adopted to ensure recovery and reduce mortality.

7. References

[1] Underhill TE, Laine FJ, George J. Diagnostic imaging of Maxillofacial infections. Oral Maxillofacial Surg Clin N Am 2003: 15; 39-49.

[2] Jones KC, Silver J, Millar WS, Mandel L. Chronic submasseteric abscess: anatomic, radiologic and pathologic features: Am J Neuroradiol 2003; 24: 1159-1163.

[3] Furuichi H, Oka M, Takenoshita Y, Kubo K, Shinohara M, Beppu K. A marked mandibular deviation caused by abscess of the pterygomandibular space. Fukuoka Igaku Zasshi 1986; 77: 373-377.

[4] Srirompstong S, Srirompotong S. Surgical emphysema following intraoral drainage of buccal space abscess. J Med Assoc Thai 2002; 85: 1314-1316.

[5] Baqain ZH, Newman L, Hyde N. How serious are oral infections? J Laryngol Otol 2004; 118: 561-565.

[6] Miller EJ Jr, Dodson TB. The risk of serious odontogenic infections in HIV-positive patients: a pilot study Oral Surg Oral Med Oral Pathol Oral Radiol Endod1998; 86: 406-409.

[7] Ugboko VI, Owotade FJ, Ajike SO, Ndukwe KC, Onipede AO. A study of orofacial bacterial infections in elderly Nigerians. SADJ 2002; 57: 391-394.

[8] Ndukwe KC, Fatusi OA, Ugboko VI. Craniocervical necrotizing fasciitis in Ile-Ife, Nigeria. Br J Oral Maxillofac Surg 2002; 40: 64-67.

[9] Hodgson TA, Rachanis CC. Oral fungal and bacterial infections in HIV-infected individuals: an overview in Africa. Oral Dis 2002; 8 Suppl 2: 80-87.

[10] Fazakerley, M. W., McGowan, P., Hardy, P. & Martin, M. V. (1993). A comparative study of cephradine, amoxycillin and phenoxymethylpenicillin in the treatment of acute dentoalveolar infection. Br Dent J 174, 359-363.[CrossRef][Medline]

[11] Flynn, T. R., Shanti, R. M. & Hayes, C. (2006). Severe odontogenic infections, part 2: prospective outcomes study. J Oral Maxillofac Surg 64, 1104–1113.[CrossRef][Medline]

[12] Fouad, A. F., Rivera, E. M. & Walton, R. E. (1996). Penicillin as a supplement in resolving the localized acute apical abscess. Oral Surg Oral Med Oral Pathol Oral Radiol Endod 81, 590–595.[CrossRef][Medline]

[13] Jimenez, Y., Bagan, J. V., Murillo, J. & Poveda, R. (2004). Odontogenic infections. Complications. Systemic manifestations. Med Oral Patol Oral Cir Bucal 9 (Suppl.), 143–147.[Medline]

[14] Kuriyama, T., Absi, E. G., Williams, D. W. & Lewis, M. A. (2005). An outcome audit of the treatment of acute dentoalveolar infection: impact of penicillin resistance. Br Dent J 198, 759–763.[CrossRef][Medline]

[15] Lewis, M. A., McGowan, D. A. & MacFarlane, T. W. (1986). Short-course high-dosage amoxycillin in the treatment of acute dento-alveolar abscess. Br Dent J 161, 299–302.[CrossRef][Medline]

[16] Lewis, M. A., Carmichael, F., MacFarlane, T. W. & Milligan, S. G. (1993). A randomised trial of co-amoxiclav (Augmentin) versus penicillin V in the treatment of acute dentoalveolar abscess. Br Dent J 175, 169–174.[CrossRef][Medline]

[17] Mangundjaja, S. & Hardjawinata, K. (1990). Clindamycin versus ampicillin in the treatment of odontogenic infections. Clin Ther 12, 242–249.[Medline]

[18] Marty-Ane, C. H., Berthet, J. P., Alric, P., Pegis, J. D., Rouviere, P. & Mary, H. (1999). Management of descending necrotizing mediastinitis: an aggressive treatment for an aggressive disease. Ann Thorac Surg 68, 212–217.[Abstract/Free Full Text]

[19] Mihos, P., Potaris, K., Gakidis, I., Papadakis, D. & Rallis, G. (2004). Management of descending necrotizing mediastinitis. J Oral Maxillofac Surg 62, 966–972.[CrossRef][Medline]

[20] Palmer, N. O. A., Martin, M. V., Pealing, R. V. & Ireland, R. S. (2000). An analysis of antibiotic prescriptions from general dental practice in England. J Antimicrob Chemother 46, 1033–1035.[Abstract/Free Full Text]

[21] Gill, Y. & Scully, C. (1990). Orofacial odontogenic infections: review of microbiology and current treatment. Oral Surg Oral Med Oral Pathol 70, 155–158.[CrossRef][Medline]

[22] Gilmore, W. C., Jacobus, N. V., Gorbach, S. L., Doku, H. C. & Tally, F. P. (1988). A prospective double-blind evaluation of penicillin versus clindamycin in the treatment of odontogenic infections. J Oral Maxillofac Surg 46, 1065–1070.[Medline]

[23] Tung-Yiu, W., Jehn-Shyun, H., Ching-Hung, C. & Hung-An, C. (2000). Cervical necrotizing fasciitis of odontogenic origin: a report of 11 cases. J Oral Maxillofac Surg 58, 1347–1352.[CrossRef][Medline]

[24] Turner Thomas, T. (1908). Ludwig's angina. An anatomical, clinical, and statistical study. Ann Surg 47, 161–163.[Medline]

[25] Wang, L. F., Kuo, W. R., Tsai, S. M. & Huang, K. J. (2003). Characterizations of life-threatening deep cervical space infections: a review of one hundred ninety-six cases. Am J Otolaryngol 24, 111–117.[CrossRef][Medline]

[26] Wang, J., Ahani, A. & Pogrel, M. A. (2005). A five-year retrospective study of odontogenic maxillofacial infections in a large urban public hospital. Int J Oral Maxillofac Surg 34, 646–649.[CrossRef][Medline].

[27] Currie WJR, Ho V. An unexpected death associated with an acute dentoalveolar abscess- Report of a case. Br J Oral Maxillofac Surg 1993; 31:296-298.

[28] Akinbami BO, Akadiri OA, Gbujie DC. Spread of orofacial infections in Port Harcourt, Nigeria. J Oral Maxillofac Surg 2010: 68; 2472-2477.

2

Aetio-Pathogenesis and Clinical Pattern of Orofacial Infections

Babatunde O. Akinbami
Department of Oral and Maxillofacial Surgery, University of Port Harcourt Teaching Hospital, Rivers State, Nigeria

1. Introduction

Microbial induced inflammatory disease in the orofacial/head and neck region which commonly arise from odontogenic tissues, should be handled with every sense of urgency, otherwise within a short period of time, they will result in acute emergency situations.[1,2] The outcome of the management of the conditions are greatly affected by the duration of the disease and extent of spread before presentation in the hospital, severity(virulence of causative organisms) of these infections as well as the presence and control of local and systemic diseases.

Odontogenic tissues include

1. Hard tooth tissue
2. Periodontium

2. Predisposing factors of orofacial infections

Local factors and systemic conditions that are associated with orofacial infections are listed below.

Local factors	Systemic factors
1. Caries, impaction, pericoronitis	Human immunodeficiency virus
2. Poor oral hygiene, periodontitis	Alcoholism
3. Trauma	Measles, chronic malaria, tuberculosis
4. Foreign body, calculi	Diabetis mellitus, hypo- and hyperthyroidism
5. Local fungal and viral infections	Liver disease, renal failure, heart failure
6. Post extraction/surgery	Blood dyscrasias
7. Irradiation	Steroid therapy
8. Failed root canal therapy	Cytotoxic drugs
9. Needle injections	Excessive antibiotics,
10. Secondary infection of tumors, cyst, fractures	Malnutrition
11. Allergic reactions	Anaemia, Sickle cell disease

In addition, low socio-economic status, level of education, neglect, self medication and ignorance are contributory factors to the development, progress and outcome of the infections[2].

3. The anatomical fascial spaces and spread of soft tissue space infection

Despite the fact that there are fasciae, muscles and bones which not only separate this region into compartments, but also serve as barriers, infections can still spread beyond the dentoalveolar tissues.[2-4]

In cases due to highly virulent organisms and also when the defense mechanism of the patient is compromised by systemic diseases, there is usually a fast spread into neighbouring, distant and intravascular spaces

- Presence of teeth and the roots below or above the attachment of the soft tissues to bone
- Density and vascularity of bone
- Presence of contiguous potential spaces in this region which are interconnected.
- Attachment of deep cervical fascia.
    - The deep cervical fascia has three divisions which separate the head and neck into compartments; the divisions include the investing (superficial), middle and deep layers. The investing layer is directly beneath the subcutaneous tissue and platysma, it is attached to the lower border of the mandible superiorly and the sternum and clavicle inferiorly.[5] The middle layer encircles central organs which include the larynx, trachea, pharynx and strap muscles, it also forms the carotid sheath anteriorly. It extends into the mediastinum to attach to the pericardium.[5]
    - The deep layer is divided into the alar fascia and the prevertebral fascia.[5] The alar fascia completes the carotid sheath posteriorly and also encloses the retropharyngeal space which extends from the base of the skull to the level of the sixth cervical vertebra. The prevertebral fascia bounds the potential prevertebral space anteriorly. It is attached to the fourth thoraxic vertebra. There is an actual space between the alar and prevertebral fascia which extends down to the diaphragm.
    - The floor of the mouth is separated from the anterior part of the neck by the mylohyoid muscle. Above this muscle is the sublingual space and this link directly with the opposite side and at the posterior aspect of the mouth it links with the submandibular space.[5] The investing layer attached to the mandible is folded into two sheaths, the upper sheath is in close proximity to the mylohyoid muscle above while the lower sheath is above the platysma, between the two is the submandibular space. The two sides of the submandibular space are separated by connective tissue septum. The body of the mandible and maxilla separates the oral cavity and the vestibule. The buccinator muscle limits the vestibule inferiorly and separates the buccal space from the vestibule.
    - Infections commonly start from the teeth or gums and these can spread via the roots or around the crowns of the teeth. It has been documented that infections from the roots of the lower anterior teeth usually spread into the sublingual space because the mylohyoid muscle attachment is below the roots, while that of the posterior teeth usually spread into the submandibular space.[6-9] Infections from the

roots of the upper anterior teeth spread into the canine fossa, except from the lateral incisors which pass more into the palatal space intraorally because of the palatal orientation of the roots,[8-10]while those from the posterior teeth spread into the buccal space. [10]

- Infections from the body of the mandible pass more through the relatively thinner lingual plate into the medial spaces while that from the body of the maxilla pass more via the relative thinner buccal plate into the lateral spaces. In addition, the ramus of the mandible serves as attachment on the outer side for masseter muscle which separates the submasseteric and supramasseteric spaces and on the inner aspect, there is attachment of medial pterygoid muscle which seperates the pterygomandibular and lateral pharyngeal spaces.[5]
- Infections from the gums around the crowns of the posterior teeth of the mandible and maxilla commonly spread to the submasseteric or pterygomandibular spaces, while that from the roots spread into the submandibular or buccal spaces and from the buccal spaces directly into the sub/supramasseteric spaces.[6-10] Also there can be spread from the submandibular space posteriorly into pterygomandibular, lateral pharyngeal and retropharyngeal spaces in the upward and downward direction.[9]
- Infections can track upwards into the infratemporal fossa between the attachments of the lateral pterygoid and temporalis muscle and into the supratemporal fossa leading to scalp abscesses. Infections can also spread into the paranasal sinuses and further into the skull, meninges, cavernose sinus/other sinuses and brain via the pterygoid plexus. Infections have also been found to spread downwards via the neck into the chest wall, mediastinum, pericardial and pleural spaces, pre and post vertebral spaces, retroperitoneal and pelvic cavities.[5-10]
- The most alarming spread of these infections is into the blood resulting in the devastating effects of septicemia which has significantly contributed to high mortality figures.[11,12]

4. Pathogenesis and spread of orofacial bone infections

Rarely does infection from the teeth, periodontium and periapical region spread beyond dentoalveolar tissue because of the vascularity and density of the basal bones. However, spread of exudates and microbes into the harversian system of bone (cancellous) below the inferior alveolar canal and beyond the maxillary sinus can occur when vascularity of the bone is reduced by excess density and cortication with aging and diseases such as osteopetrosis.

Lacunae space connections between the alveolar bone and basal bone below the inferior alveolar canal as well as connections with trabeculae bone around the maxillary sinuses, enhance spread into the whole mandible or maxilla especially in immunocompromised patients.

Increased pressure within the bone compromises vascularity causing ischeamia, necrosis of both trabeculae and lamella bone, and sequestra formation. Exudates escape through the Volkmann's canal into the subperiosteal space, stripping the periosteum. Inflammatory periosteal reaction causes laying down and formation of new bone (involucrum) around the sequestrum.

In the sclerotic, subperiosteatis ossificans types, chronic inflammation due to low grade infections (less virulent organisms) induces more granulation tissue formation, organisation of fibrous tissue, consolidation and later dystrophic calcification.

5. Classification of orofacial soft tissue space infections

Infections can be classified based not only on the type of organisms, it can also be

Based on the site/space involved

- Spaces related to the mandible include
  Submandibular,
  Sublingual and
  Submental spaces
  Sub- , intra- and supramasseteric,
  Pterygomandibular,
  Lateral pharyngeal and
  Infratemporal spaces[2].
- Bilateral submandibular, sublingual and submental spaces are involved in Ludwig's angina. The incidence of Ludwig's angina has declined over the years with the advent of antibiotics[1] and only 5 cases were recorded in the study of Akinbami 2010.

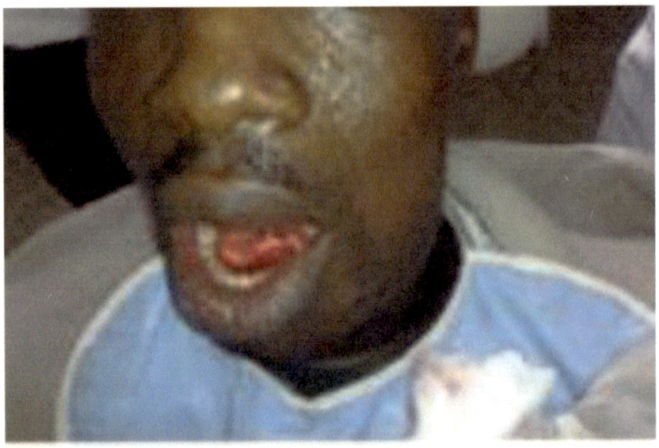

Fig. 1.

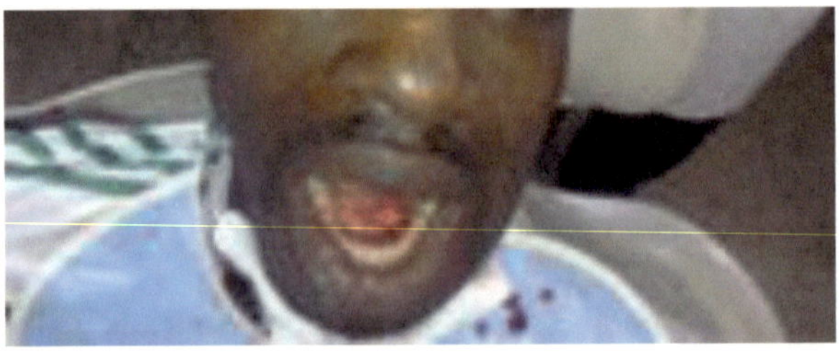

Fig. 2.

Fig. 1 and 2 show Pre-operative and Post-operative Photographs of a 31-year-old patient treated for Ludwig's angina, submasseteric absess and buccal space abscess

- Spaces related to the maxilla
  Soft tissue space infections related to the maxilla and middle third of the face include
  Canine fossa abscess, and
  Buccal space infections
  Infection can be localized in a single space and can also spread to involve multiple spaces.

Based on the pattern/direction

- Below or above the floor of the mouth
- Below or above the palate

Based on the extent of spread

- Dentoalveolar tissues e.g. periapical, periodontium, alveolar bone, in rare cases to the basal bone (osteomyelitis)
- Soft tissue space around the jaws
- Space beyond the jaws e.g. neck, orbit, brain/skull,
- Distant sites; chest/pleura space, heart-endocardium, myocardium and pericardium, diaphragm, vertebra , abdomen and pelvis.

6. Classification of orofacial bone infections

Infections affecting the hard tissues can either be in the form of acute or chronic dentoalveolar abscess and osteomyelitis.

Osteomyelitis is a more severe bone infection and it can be classified into suppurative or sclerosing;

- Acute suppurative osteomyelitis
- Chronic suppurative osteomyelitis,
- Focal sclerosing osteomyelitis (Garre's osteomyelitis)
- Diffuse sclerosing osteomyelitis.

It can also be classified based on the site as

- Intramedullary osteomyelitis,
- Cortical osteomyelitis
- Acute and
- Chronic periostitis
- Subperiostitis ossificans also described by Garre's
- Refractory osteomyelitis

7. Microbial etiology of orofacial infections

The aetiologies of bone, soft tissue and tissue space infections are:

Non-specific bacteria and specific organisms such as viral, fungi, tuberculosis, syphilis and salmonella species[9].

Other factors include, irradiation, chemicals like mercury and phosphorus.[2,4]

Most bacteria induce inflammation by producing various antigens e.g, M protein antigen encoded by *emm* - like gene.

Orofacial infections are caused and can be classified based on the causative organisms

- Non specific (acute bacterial; aerobic, anaerobic, mixed) Causative organisms that have been incriminated for these non-specific infections are mixed in nature, that is, facultative anaerobic, strict anaerobic and aerobic organisms.
- Specific (chronic bacterial infection, fungal, viral) Specific infections are caused by organisms like *tuberculosis, syphilis, actinomycosis and viral* organism[s4].

Orofacial infections are usually polymicrobial comprising

- Facultative anaerobes, such as non-heamolytic Streptococci viridans group and heamolytic Streptococci anginosus group especially, Group A beta hemolytic, as well as Group C and Group G.
- Both C and G are occasionally obtained from throat cultures and very responsive to the new antibiotic, Linezolid (Zyvox) of the oxazolidinone class, which blocks protein synthesis by preventing translation. It binds the 23s ribosomal RNA and then hinders formation of functional 70s RNA from 50s RNA subspecies.
- And predominantly strict anaerobes, such as anaerobic cocci, Prevotella and Fusobacterium species.
- Aerobic organisms like Pseudomonas sp, Proteus sp., and Klebsiella sp. Many of them are actually nosocomial (hospital acquired) organisms . These are enterobacteria that are recently found in orofacial infections.

The use of non-culture techniques has expanded our insight into the microbial diversity of the causative agents, identifying such organisms as Treponema species and anaerobic Gram-positive rods such as Bulleidia extructa, Cryptobacterium curtum and Mogibacterium timidum.

- Efforts to identify the causative pathogens involved in the development of the dental abscess have in the past been hampered by inappropriate methods of sampling. The ideal clinical sample from an acute dental abscess is an aspirate through intact mucosa disinfected by an appropriate antiseptic mouthwash or swab, e.g. chlorhexidine, although some researchers have sampled purulent exudates from within infected canals (Lewis et al., 1990; Chavez de Paz Villanueva, 2002). This will reduce contamination from the normal oral flora. Previous studies using swabs of purulent material have demonstrated poor recovery of strict anaerobes and low mean numbers of isolates per sample (range 1.0–1.6) (Lewis et al., 1990).
- Pure cultures from an acute dental abscess are unusual (Reader et al., 1994), and mixed aerobic infections are also uncommon, accounting for 6 % of abscesses (Goumas et al., 1997). Dental abscesses caused solely by strict anaerobes occur in approximately 20 % of cases although there is a wide range depending on recovery conditions (6–63 %) (Brook et al., 1991; Gorbach et al., 1991; Goumas et al., 1997; Khemaleelakul et al., 2002).

- A complex mix of strict anaerobes and facultative anaerobes accounts for most infections (59–75 %), which can prove challenging to non-specialist microbiology laboratories (Gorbach et al., 1991; Goumas et al., 1997; Kuriyama et al., 2000a). In mixed infections, strict anaerobes outnumber facultatives by a ratio which varies between 1.5: 1 to 3 : 1, again depending on the recovery and culture conditions (Baumgartner & Xia, 2003; Khemaleelakul et al., 2002; Kulekci et al., 1996; Lewis et al., 1993; Roche & Yoshimori, 1997; Sakamoto et al., 1998). The mean number of species recovered by culture from dentoalveolar aspirates is 4 with a range of between 1 and 7.5 (Fazakerley et al., 1993; Khemaleelakul et al., 2002; Reader et al., 1994).

Facultative anaerobes

The most commonly found facultative anaerobes belong to the viridans group streptococci and the anginosus group streptococci.

- The viridans group streptococci comprise the mitis group, oralis group, salivarius group, sanguinis group and the mutans group (Facklam, 2002).
- The anginosus group (formerly referred to as 'Streptococcus milleri' or Streptococcus anginosus) has also been identified and reported with varying degrees of accuracy ranging. These are alpha, beta and gamma haemolytic streptococci.

Historically, Staphylococcus species have not been considered members of the oral flora or to play a major role in the pathogenesis of oral infections. However, a number of more recent studies have indicated that both 'methiccilin sensitive and resistant' staphylococci may indeed be a more frequent colonizer of the oral tissues than previously thought.

Interestingly, Staphylococcus aureus has been reported to occur more frequently in severe dental abscesses from children (Brook et al., 1991; Coticchia et al., 2004; Coulthard & Isaacs, 1991; Dodson et al., 1989; Tan et al., 2001). Recovery rates of coagulase-negative strains of staphylococci (usually reported as Staphylococcus epidermidis) are generally higher with figures ranging from 4 to 65 % (Gorbach et al., 1991; Goumas et al., 1997; Khemaleelakul et al., 2002; Kuriyama et al., 2002b; Lewis et al., 1995; Mangundjaja & Hardjawinata, 1990; Sakamoto et al., 1998; Storoe et al., 2001). Staphylococcus species may also be associated with refractory infections not responding to endodontic treatment (Reader et al., 1994).

Strict Anaerobes

Similar difficulties exist for cross-study comparisons of identification and prevalence of strict anaerobes. The most commonly isolated genera include

- Anaerobic streptococci, Fusobacterium species and
- Black-pigmented anaerobes such as Prevotella and Porphyromonas species (Sundqvist et al., 1989).

The nomenclature and recent changes in taxonomy have complicated the comparison of more recent studies with older studies due to the renaming of several species, specifically the Prevotella, Bacteroides and Porphyromonas species. An important group of pathogens that has undergone much in the way of taxonomic rearrangement, often referred to as the 'oral Bacteroides' and black-pigmenting anaerobes group, has been reclassified.

The Bacteroides species have been divided into the

- saccharolytic genus Prevotella and the asaccharolytic genus Porphyromonas.

The genus Bacteroides has been restricted to the

- fermentative Bacteroides fragilis and its closely related species.

B. fragilis, a more common isolate from intra-abdominal infections, which has only infrequently been reported from acute dentoalveolar infections, is not regarded as an oral commensal.

The member of the Bacteroides genus most likely to be recovered from an acute dental abscess is Bacteroides forsythus (now transferred to a new genus as Tannerella forsythia (Gomes et al., 2006).

The most commonly reported anaerobic Gram-negative bacilli from acute dentoalveolar infections are species from the

- pigmented Prevotella intermedia (comprising Prevotella intermedia, Prevotella nigrescens and Prevotella pallens),
- Porphyromonas endodontalis and Porphyromonas gingivalis (Jacinto et al., 2006).

The Prevotella species are the most frequent isolates, found in

- 10–87 % of dentoalveolar abscesses (Baumgartner et al., 2004; Fazakerley et al., 1993; Kolokotronis, 1999; Kulekci et al., 1996; Kuriyama et al., 2005; Lewis et al., 1993; Riggio et al., 2006; Roche & Yoshimori, 1997; Sakamoto et al., 1998; Siqueira et al., 2001b, d; Wade et al., 1994).

The genus Fusobacterium is frequently reported in infections of the head and neck with reports indicating that Fusobacterium species can be detected in up to 52 % of specimens (Gill & Scully, 1990; Gilmore et al., 1988; Gorbach et al., 1991; Goumas et al., 1997; Kulekci et al., 1996; Kuriyama et al., 2000a, b, 2005, 2006; Lewis et al., 1993; Mangundjaja & Hardjawinata, 1990; Sakamoto et al., 1998; Wade et al., 1994).

- Taxonomy and nomenclature of the genus Fusobacterium also cause difficulties in comparisons across studies. Within the human oral flora,
- Fusobacterium periodonticum and Fusobacterium nucleatum (which includes subsp. nucleatum, subsp. polymorphum, subsp. animalis, subsp. vincentii and subsp. fusiforme) are frequently detected with F. nucleatum recovered most frequently from the acute dental abscess (Dzink et al., 1990; Chavez de Paz Villanueva, 2002; Sassone et al., 2008).
- Studies utilizing non-culture techniques for analysis of the dental abscess for the presence of F. nucleatum have reported a prevalence of 73 % (Baumgartner et al., 2004).

The Clostridia are infrequently reported from odontogenic infections either as a sole pathogen or as part of the abscess flora. Workers have recovered

- Clostridium species from 2–20 % of specimens (Gorbach et al., 1991; Goumas et al., 1997; Khemaleelakul et al., 2002; Roche & Yoshimori, 1997). Where speciated, these isolates have included
- Clostridium hastiforme
- Clostridium histolyticum

- Clostridium perfringens
- Clostridium subterminale and
- Clostridium clostridioforme (Khemaleelakul et al., 2002; Roche & Yoshimori, 1997).

Although other Clostridium species such as Clostridium sporogenes, Clostridium bifermentans, Clostridium botulinum, 'Clostridium oedomatiens' and 'Clostridium welchii' have been recovered from carious dentine, they appear to be infrequent pathogens in the oral cavity (Van Reenan & Coogan, 1970).

- Analysis of the microflora of the acute dental abscess using molecular biological techniques. Close attention to specimen collection and processing on selective and non-selective agars under appropriate atmospheric conditions has improved the routine diagnostic yield from acute dental abscesses. However, despite meticulous attention to detail, it is apparent that many genera of bacteria have yet to be cultured from many infectious diseases including the acute dental abscess (Siqueira & Rocas, 2005).
- The use of culture-independent or molecular diagnostic techniques has expanded our insight into the microbial ecology of the dental abscess. Genetic methods of identification are now reliable with 16S rRNA gene sequencing frequently being used for research purposes. Broadly speaking, the molecular analysis may take one of two approaches.
- Firstly, the use of molecular cloning and sequencing techniques to identify uncultivable micro-organisms using 16s rRNA or rDNA has led to the identification of several novel species (Dymock et al., 1996).
- Secondly, is the use of Polymerase Chain Reaction (PCR) or DNA–DNA hybridization chequerboard techniques (Siqueira et al., 2001d, 2002a) and more recently 16S rRNA gene sequencing and species-specific primers searching for the presence of specific microbes (Dymock et al., 1996; Riggio et al., 2006; Rocas & Siqueira, 2005; Sakamoto et al., 2006; Siqueira et al., 2001b, c, 2002b, 2003). There is higher prevalence of more fastidious organisms such as Treponema species in the acute dental abscess with this second approach.

Treponema species are strictly anaerobic, motile, helically shaped bacteria. Within the oral cavity they are more usually associated with diseases of the periodontium. There are a number of different species described from the oral cavity including

- Treponema amylovorum
- Treponema denticola
- Treponema maltophilum
- Treponema medium
- Treponema pectinovorum
- Treponema socranskii and
- Treponema vincentii (Chan & McLaughlin, 2000).
    - The treponemes are difficult to cultivate and differentiate and only T. denticola, T. pectinovorum, T. socranskii and 'T. vincentii' have been readily cultivated. Recent work using PCR detection has indicated a surprisingly high prevalence of Treponema species within the acute dental abscess. Siqueira & Rocas (2004c) found that T. denticola was present in up to 79 % of dental abscesses, with lower detection rates reported by other workers (Baumgartner et al., 2003; Siqueira et al., 2001a, c; Gomes et al., 2006; Cavrini et al., 2008).

- Other Treponema species were found in lower numbers, including T. socranskii (in 26 % of aspirates), T. pectinovorum (14–21 % of aspirates), T. amylovorum (16 % of aspirates) and T.medium (5 % of aspirates). Other species such as Treponema lecithinolyticum, 'T. vincentii' and T. maltophilum were not detected.

Improvements in sampling, culture and identification have led to a greater insight into the diversity of the microbial flora in an acute dental abscess. This has resulted in the reporting of micro-organisms which are probably more accurately described as 'unfamiliar' rather than 'new' implying their recent appearance.

These include members of the genus Atopobium

- (Gram-positive strictly anaerobic coccobacilli), for example Atopobium parvulum and Atopobium rimae.
- Anaerobic Gram-positive rods include Bulleidia extructa, Cryptobacterium curtum,
- Eubacterium sulci, Mogibacterium timidum and Mogibacterium vescum (Sakamoto et al., 2006), Pseudoramibacter alactolyticus and Slakia exigua (Siqueira & Rocas, 2003c).

Other unfamiliar species include anaerobic Gram-negative rods such as

- Filifactor alocis (Siqueira & Rocas, 2003a, 2004b; Gomes et al., 2006) and
- Dialister pneumosintes (Siqueira et al., 2005; Siqueira & Rocas, 2003b, 2004b).
- Centipeda periodontii and Selenomonas sputigena are multi-flagellated, motile, anaerobic, Gram-negative rods also found recently in the acute dental abscess (Siqueira & Rocas, 2004a).
- Catonella morbi, a Gram-negative anaerobe formerly known as Bacteroides D42, was found in 16 % of 19 aspirates, and Granulicatella adiacens, a facultative anaerobic Gram-positive coccus formerly known as nutritionally variant streptococci, was present in 11 % of 19 aspirates (Rocas & Siqueira, 2005; Siqueira & Rocas, 2006).
  - The detection of these unfamiliar species has opened up a whole new area for possible study into the virulence factors possessed by these bacteria and their relative influence on the pathogenesis of the acute dental abscess and interactions with more commonly isolated and better understood pathogens. These techniques are not without their limitations and meticulous asepsis is required throughout the sampling and analysis procedure to avoid contamination due to the sensitivity of these methods.
  - Furthermore, until recently these techniques could only give semiquantitative analysis of aspirates and indeed some papers cited above can only show the presence or absence of the species in question. This will improve with the advent of quantitative real-time PCR. The use of species-specific primers targeting the 16S rRNA gene or similar is also limited by the fact that they cannot distinguish between transcriptionally active viable cells and those non-vital bystanders. Advanced molecular techniques using reverse transcriptase are finding methods of overcoming these limitations currently. Also, molecular techniques provide little information to guide the clinician in the choice of antibiotic required.

8. Evaluation of orofacial soft tissue space infections

Infections within the soft tissue spaces constitute about 61% of all orofacial infections and they are commoner in males than females in both adult and pediatric age groups[16]

Histories of complains such as

- Toothache, pain from any of the site precede that of
  - Swelling
  - Cellulites in these spaces is characterized by severe pain and marked trismus
  - Swelling is more prominent in supramasseteric space than submasseteric space,
  - Trismus is marked in the pterygomandibular, submasseteric and infratemporal spaces[3-5]
  - Pain and swelling manifest more intraorally in pterygomandibular and lateral pharyngeal space infections[6-10]
  - Dypsnea and Stridor
  - Difficulty in lying supine; most patients want to sit up, in attempt to get enough breath
  - Systemic signs: Features of systemic spread are fever, chills, rigors, anorexia, nausea

Examine

- Site, size and extent of swelling and restriction in mouth opening; e.g.,
  Infections in the lateral pharyngeal space spread down to the posterior triangle as well as underneath and around the sternomastoid muscle. Buccal space infections are located more anteriorly and extraorally[2]. Infratemporal cellulitis spread more towards the temporal region
- Offending tooth; caries, fracture, failed crown/root filling, tenderness to percussion, loss of vitality, inflammed gingiva, recession, pockets.
- Associated discharge from the gingiva sulci
- Paraesthesia/anaesthesia
- Vital signs: Temperature, pulse rate, respiratory rate. Features of systemic spread are raised temperature, increased pulse rate and increasing respiratory rate.
- Furuichi *et al.* reported gross mandibular deviation in a case pterygomandibular abscess.[9]

9. Evaluation of orofacial bone infections

Dentoalveolar abscess is the commonest bone infection usually secondary to local factors and it is common in all age groups with incidence of 21.7%. Osteomyelitis is about 8.7% and occurs more in the middle age and elderly due to reduced vascularity and increased bone density of bone with age. Similarly, the disease also occur more in the mandible than maxilla[2]. However, acute maxillitis of the newborn is a disease that is due to the primary infection opthalmia neonatarium acquired from organisms in the birth canal[2].

Dento-alveolar abscess present with

- moderate to severe pain

- moderate swelling of the alveolus more prominent on the buccal side
- tenderness to percussion of the affected teeth
- usually no altered sensation
- mild to moderate mobility of teeth
- occasionally pus discharge from the sulci
- rarely, there may be intraoral sinus formation in chronic cases

Acute osteomyelitis manifests with

- severe systemic signs
- deep-seated pain in the bone
- pus discharge from the gingival sulci
- moderate bone swelling, welling of the teeth
- severe tenderness to percussion and
- absent sensations (anaesthesia)

Chronic osteomyelitis present with

- a dull pain
- moderate / large bony hard swellings
- altered sensations (paraesthesia)
- persistent discharging extraoral sinuses and
- new bone formation. Formation of involucrum around the sequestrum
    - There have been controversies over the origin and aetiology of diffuse sclerosing osteomyelitis. Some authors believe that it is due to organisms like *propionibacterium acne and peptostreptococcus intermedius* found in the deep pockets associated with generalized periodontitis. Others believe that it may be part of a bone, joint and skin {SAPHO; synovitis, acne, pustulosis, hyperostosis and osteitis} syndrome probably due to allergic or autoimmune reaction in the periosteum[7]. Based on this fact, it has been found that corticosteroids have been useful in its management with or without prolonged antibiotic therapy and decortications

10. Microbiology

Microscopy/Culture/Sensitivity

Different types of agars for culture and sensitivity

- Gram staining techniques for microscopy and identification of organisms
- Blood agar culture: MacKonchey media
- Antibiotic laden vancomycin-kanamycin agar
- Bile agar

Anaerobic culture

- Thioglycolate agar
- Cooked meat broth agar

Sensitivity Test

- Disk diffusion sensitivity tests for antibiotics sensitivity

11. Chemical pathology

- Evaluation for systemic factors, , fasting blood sugar, Electrolyte/urea/cretinine

12. Virology and immunology

- Retroviral screening

13. Hematology

- Packed cell volume
- White blood count; total and differential,
- Blood films and bone marrow aspirates to rule out leukemia, polycythemia, aplastic anaemia
- Erythrocyte sedimentation rate

14. References

[1] Shafer WG. Infectious diseases. In: Hine MK, Levy BM, eds. A textbook of oral pathology. 3rd ed. Philadelphia, USA: WB Saunder's Company, 1974:309-355.
[2] Killey HC, Kay LW. Orofacial infections. In: Seward GR, Harris M, McGowan DA, eds. An outline of oral surgery Part Two. 4th ed. Oxford, Great Britain: Reed educational and professional publishing limited, 1989:310- 330.
[3] Contran RS. Infectious diseases. In: Kumar V, Collin Y, eds. Pathologic basis of disease. 6th ed. London, WB Saunders Company 1999:169- 193.
[4] Soames JV. Pathological basis of infection. In: Southam JC, ed. Textbook of oral pathology. 3rd ed. New York: Oxford University Press, 1995:245-265.
[5] Sinnatamby R. Anatomy of the Head and Neck region. In: Last RJ, ed. Regional and applied anatomy. 9th ed. Philadelphia: Churchill Livingstone 1998:456-478.
[6] Cawson RA. Management of infectious diseases In Cawson RA ed. Essentials of oral pathology and oral medicine. 1st ed. London: Micheal Parkinson 1981:88-95.
[7] Siegert R. Ultrasonography of inflammatory soft tissue swellings of the head and neck region. J Oral Maxillofac Surg 1987;45:842-846.
[8] Jones KC, Silver J, Millar WS, Mandel L. Chronic submasseteric abscess: anatomic, radiologic and pathologic features: Am J Neuroradiol 2003;24: 1159-1163.
[9] Furuichi H, Oka M, Takenoshita Y, Kubo K, Shinohara M, Beppu K. A marked mandibular deviation caused by abscess of the pterygomandibular space. Fukuoka Igaku Zasshi 1986;77:373-377.
[10] Srirompstong S, Srirompotong S. Surgical emphysema following intraoral drainage of buccal space abscess. J Med Assoc Thai 2002;85: 1314-1316.
[11] Baqain ZH, Newman L, Hyde N. How serious are oral infections? J Laryngol Otol 2004;118:561-565.

[12] Miller EJ Jr, Dodson TB. The risk of serious odontogenic infections in HIV-positive patients: a pilot study. Oral Surg Oral Med Oral Pathol Oral Radiol Endod 1998;86:406-409.

[13] Ugboko VI, Owotade FJ, Ajike SO, Ndukwe KC, Onipede AO. A study of orofacial bacterial infections in elderly Nigerians. SADJ 2002;57:391-394.

[14] Ndukwe KC, Fatusi OA, Ugboko VI. Craniocervical necrotizing fasciitis in Ile-Ife, Nigeria. Br J Oral Maxillofac Surg 2002;40:64-67.

[15] Hodgson TA, Rachanis CC. Oral fungal and bacterial infections in HIV-infected individuals: an overview in Africa. Oral Dis 2002;8(Suppl 2):80-87.

[16] Akinbami BO. Factors associated with orofacial infections. Port Harcourt Medical Journal 2009;3:199-206.

[17] Iwahara K, Kuriyama T, Shimura S, Williams DW, Yanagisawa M, Nakagawa K, Karasawa T. Detection of cfx a and cfxA2, the ß-lactamase genes of Prevotella spp. in clinical samples of dentoalveolar infection by real-time PCR. Journal of Clinical Microbiology 2006;44:172-176

[18] Sandor GK, Low DE, Judd PL, Davidson RJ. Antimicrobial treatment options in the management of odontogenic infections. J Can. Dent Assoc 1998;64:508-514.

[19] Parker MI, Khateery SM. A retrospective analysis of orofacial infection requiring hospitalization in AL Madinah, Saudi Arabia. Saudi Dental Journal 2001;13:96-100.

[20] Heimdahl A, Nord CE. Treatment of orofacial infections of odontogenic origin. Scand J Infect Dis 1989;46(Suppl):101-105.

[21] Sandor GKB, Low DE, Judd PL, Davidson RJ. Antimicrobial treatment options in the management of odontogenic infections. J Canad Dent Asso 1998;64:508-514.

[22] Greenberg RN, James RB, Marier RL. Microbiologic and antibiotic aspects of infections in the Oral and Maxillofacial region. J Oral Surg 1979;37:873-884.

[23] Moenning JE, Nelson CL, Kohler RB. The microbiology and chemotherapy of odontogenic infections. J Oral Maxillofac Surg 1989; 47:976982.

[24] Baker KA, Fotos PG. The management of odontogenic infections. A rationale for appropriate chemotherapy. Dent Clin North Am 1994; 36:689-706.

[25] Sands T, Pynn BR, Katsikeris N. Odontogenic infections: Microbiology, antibiotics and management. Oral Health 1995;85:11-28.

[26] Sands T, Pynn BR. Odontogenic infections. Univ Tufts Dent J 1995;32-33.

[27] Haug RH, Hoffman MJ, Indresano AT. An epidemiological and anatomical survey of odontogenic infections. J Oral Maxillofac Surg 1991;47:976-980.

[28] Hunt DE, King TJ, Fuller GE. Antibiotic susceptibility of bacteria isolated from oral infections. J Oral Surg 1978;36:527.

[29] Peters ES, Fong Brian, Wormuth DW, Sonis ST. Risk factors affecting hospital length of stay in patients with odontogenic maxillofacial infections. J Oral Maxillofac Surg 1996;54:1386-1391.

[30] Van Reenan, J. F. & Coogan, M. M. (1970). Clostridia isolated from human mouths. ArchOral Biol 15, 845–848.[CrossRef][Medline]

[31] Bonapart IE, Stevens HPJD, Kerver AJH, Rietveld AP. Rare complications of an odontogenic abscess; Mediastinitis, Thoracic empyema and Cardiac Tamponade. J Oral Maxillofac Surg 1995;53:610-613.

[32] Robertson D. and Smith AJ (2009). The microbiology of the acute dental abscess. Journal of Medical Microbiology 58 (2): 155-172
[33] Baumgartner, J. C., Khemaleelakul, S. U. & Xia, T. (2003). Identification of spirochetes (treponemes) in endodontic infections. J Endod 29, 794–797.[Medline]
[34] Baumgartner, J. C., Siqueira, J. F., Jr, Xia, T. & Rocas, I. N. (2004). Geographical differences in bacteria detected in endodontic infections using polymerase chain reaction. J Endod 30, 141–144.[Medline]
[35] Brook, I. (1987). Microbiology of retropharyngeal abscesses in children. Am J Dis Child 141, 202–204.[Abstract/Free Full Text]
[36] Brook, I., Frazier, E. H. & Gher, M. E. (1991). Aerobic and anaerobic microbiology of periapical abscess. Oral Microbiol Immunol 6, 123–125.[Medline]
[37] Cavrini, F., Pirani, C., Foschi, F., Montebugnoli, L., Sambri, V. & Prati, C. (2008). Detection of Treponema denticola in root canal systems in primary and secondary endodontic infections. A correlation with clinical symptoms. New Microbiol 31, 67–73.[Medline]
[38] Chan, E. C. & McLaughlin, R. (2000). Taxonomy and virulence of oral spirochetes. Oral Microbiol Immunol 15, 1–9.[CrossRef][Medline]
[39] Chavez de Paz Villanueva, L. E. (2002). Fusobacterium nucleatum in endodontic flare-ups. Oral Surg Oral Med Oral Pathol Oral Radiol Endod 93, 179–183.[CrossRef][Medline]
[40] Dymock, D., Weightman, A. J., Scully, C. & Wade, W. G. (1996). Molecular analysis of microflora associated with dentoalveolar abscesses. J Clin Microbiol 34, 537–542.[Abstract]
[41] Gomes, B. P., Jacinto, R. C., Pinheiro, E. T., Sousa, E. L., Zaia, A. A., Ferraz, C. C. & Souza-Filho, F. J. (2006). Molecular analysis of Filifactor alocis, Tannerella forsythia, and Treponema denticola associated with primary endodontic infections and failed endodontic treatment. J Endod 32, 937–940.[CrossRef][Medline]
[42] Gorbach, S. L., Gilmore, W. C., Jacobus, N. V., Doku, H. C. & Tally, F. P. (1991). Microbiology and antibiotic resistance in odontogenic infections. Ann Otol Rhinol Laryngol Suppl 154, 40–42.[Medline]
[43] Goumas, P. D., Naxakis, S. S., Papavasiliou, D. A., Moschovakis, E. D., Tsintsos, S. J. & Skoutelis, A. (1997). Periapical abscesses: causal bacteria and antibiotic sensitivity. J Chemother 9, 415–419.[Medline]
[44] Kulekci, G., Inanc, D., Kocak, H., Kasapoglu, C. & Gumru, O. Z. (1996). Bacteriology of dentoalveolar abscesses in patients who have received empirical antibiotic therapy. Clin Infect Dis 23 (Suppl. 1), S51–S53.[Medline]
[45] Kuriyama, T., Karasawa, T., Nakagawa, K., Yamamoto, E. & Nakamura, S. (2001). Incidence of beta-lactamase production and antimicrobial susceptibility of anaerobic gram-negative rods isolated from pus specimens of orofacial odontogenic infections. Oral Microbiol Immunol 16, 10–15.[CrossRef][Medline]
[46] Siqueira, J. F., Jr & Rocas, I. N. (2004b). Simultaneous detection of Dialister pneumosintes and Filifactor alocis in endodontic infections by 16S rDNA-directed multiplex PCR. J Endod 30, 851–854.[CrossRef][Medline]

[47] Siqueira, J. F., Jr & Rocas, I. N. (2004c). Treponema species associated with abscesses of endodontic origin. Oral Microbiol Immunol 19, 336-339.[CrossRef][Medline]

[48] Siqueira, J. F., Jr, Rocas, I. N., Favieri, A., Oliveira, J. C. & Santos, K. R. (2001c). Polymerase chain reaction detection of Treponema denticola in endodontic infections within root canals. Int Endod J 34, 280-284.[CrossRef][Medline]

[49] Siqueira, J. F., Rocas, I. N., De Uzeda, M., Colombo, A. P. & Santos, K. R. (2002a). Comparison of 16S rDNA-based PCR and checkerboard DNA-DNA hybridisation for detection of selected endodontic pathogens. J Med Microbiol 51, 1090-1096.[Abstract/Free Full Text]

[50] Storoe, W., Haug, R. H. & Lillich, T. T. (2001). The changing face of odontogenic infections. Oral Maxillofac Surg 59, 739-748.[CrossRef][Medline].

3

The Forearm Flap – Indications, Appropriate Selection, Complications and Functional Outcome

Raphael Ciuman and Philipp Dost
Department of Otorhinolaryngology, Marienhospital Gelsenkirchen, Gelsenkirchen, Germany

1. Introduction

A correct indication and specific knowledege in planning and harvesting free transplants are needed to minimize morbidity and maximize quality of life (QOL). Since the introduction of microvascular surgery in the 1970s, continuous surgical efforts and research were made to optimize the techniques. Consequently, there exist distinct technical modifications and alternatives that give the surgeon the possibility of adequate technique and flap-design selection dependent on the patient and situation. In the 1990s, the free forearm flap became the most utilised technique for free tissue transfer in the head and neck, with success rates of over 90% (Soutar & McGreagor, 1986, Swanson et al., 1990). The forearm flap was described by Yang and colleagues in 1981 for the first time and has become one of the most used transplants for reconstruction in the head and neck and a widely used transplant for other indications as well. Various complications and functional impairments at the donor site have been reported so far which are presented together with techniques to minimize them, and together with the characteristics, indications and design options of this flap.

2. Historical description

In 1978, Yang Guofan und Gao Yuzhi harvested a fasciocutaneous radial free flap in the Shenyang Military Hospital for the first time. This transplant got the nickname 'Chinese flap' and became the standard transplant for many indications. In 1981, they described a study of 60 patients with a single transplant loss only. Mühlbauer et al. (1982) were the first who reported upon this transplant outside of China. Stock and contributors raised an innervated flap in 1981 and in 1983, Biemer and Stock utilised an osteocutaneous pedicled transplant for thumb reconstruction. Lovie reported upon an ulnar-based forearm flap in 1984 that was classified as alternative to avoid vascular complications at the donor site by Dost and Rudofsky (1993) (Figure 1). Soutar (1983) proposed the forearm flap for reconstruction of the oral cavity, and thereafter the flap became the most utilised technique for intraoral reconstruction. Partecke et al. described a fat fascia only transplant in 1986 which results in a cosmetic appealing scar line. The defect at the recipient site was covered with a split-thickness graft. Finally, tendons and muscles were included in the transplant as well

(Cavanagh et al., 1991). To improve the donor site morbidity, Webster and Robinson (1995) as well as S.C. Chang et al. (1996) described a suprafascial raised forearm flap in the 1990s but there were no differences demonstrable concerning the sensory outcome. Wolff and colleagues (1995) described a prefabricated fascial-split-thickness flap, and Rath and contributors (1997) widened the technical varieties by introducing a prelaminated fasciomucosal flap that was raised after six weeks. Interesting are the work of Costa and colleagues (1993) who used silicon moulds, silicone tubes and split-thickness grafts to reconstruct mouth, nose or ear, and the work of Pribaz und Fine (1994) who provided auricular cartilage into the flap to reconstruct the nose. Besides titanium mesh together with a free forearm flap can be used for reconstruction in the head and neck (Hashikawa et al., 2006; Kubo et al., 2009).

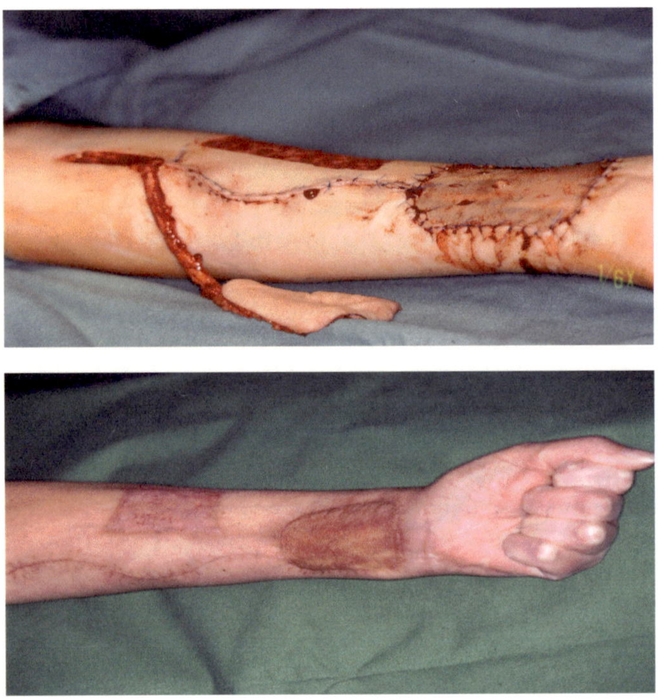

Fig. 1. The ulnar forearm free flap after harvesting and covering the donor defect with split-thickness skin graft intraoperative and three months later

To choose the functional and aesthetic most adequate and for the patient least stressful transplant, all designs fasciocutaneous/cutaneous, musculocutaneous/muscle, osteocutaneous/osteomusculocutaneous should be considered. Musculocutaneous flaps are superior to fasciocutaneous flaps for deep, poor vascularized and infected defects. Table 1 summarizes the characteristics and indications for the most adequate forearm flap designs.

transplant design	**characteristics**	**indications**
faciocutaneous transplant	*standard transplant with the most indications and described recipient sites*	defects of the oral cavity; a modeling in the glossoalveolaris sulcus is easier when the mandible is preserved tongue reconstruction for defects > 50%; superficial tongue defects, especially the oral part pharynx reconstruction; also when a muscle flap was lost before middle-sized defects of the skull base defects of the midface and orbit oronasel fistulas associated with palate defects pretibial defects hand- and arm reconstruction heel defects
suprafascially elevated transplant	*the remaining fascia decreases wound healing and functional impairment* *improved cosmetic result , but not improved sensory outcome*	defects of the oral cavity
with split-thickness skin prefabricated transplant	*improved cosmetic result at the forearm* *about 10-15% shrinking at the recipient site* *prolonged therapy*	back of the hand, because of a declined tendency for oedema and impaired function compared to the palm intraoral defects
prelaminated fasciomucosal transplant	*high compatibility at the recipient site* *prevention of xerostomia* *no reepitheliation and scar tissue formation at the recipient site* *silicon sheets allow an expansion of about 30-50%* *prolonged therapy*	defects of the oral cavity
innervated transplant	*improved sensory potency* *prevention of aspiration*	tongue reconstruction; especially the oral part poor sensory potency, e.g. after trigeminus resection trauma with nerve damage palm and sole penile and urethral construction

transplant design	characteristics	indications
osteocutaneous transplant	*bone up to a length of 12 cm is harvestable*	mandibular reconstruction for defects of up to 9 cm length; especially defects of the ramus and those with small bone and large soft-tissue defects
teno-musculocutaneous transplant	*robust transplant, but increased donor site morbidity* *harvesting a single muscle, in most cases the brachioradialis muscle, is possible as well*	tongue reconstruction reconstruction of the floor of the mouth external defects infection, e.g. osteomyelitis hand and elbow defects
fat-fascia transplant	*highly vascularized tissue* *cosmetic and functional result at the donor site* *not the adequate transplant for exposed recipient sites, when coverage with split-thickness graft is necessary*	transplant to improve filling and sliding; especially for the back of the hand hand and elbow oral cavity
pedicled transplant	*length of the incision is reduced* *possibility of local anesthesia* *but a flap fixation for about 14 days is necessary*	defects of the hand or arm skin defects

Table 1. Aspects of selecting the adequate transplant design

3. Important anatomical variations

Important anatomical variations in regards with the free forearm flap transfer were reported, and should be described briefly. The raised forearm flap area should not extend beyond the antecubital fossa and the radial or ulnar borders to avoid complications and sensory impairment. Yang et al. (1981) described a forearm flap of 35x15 cm, but the dimensions of the forearm transplant are limited by the bifurcation of the forearm arteries at the level of the antecubital fossa.

Both, the radial and the ulnar artery participate in the blood supply of the palmar arches but show in only 27-35% equal supply to the hand and fingers (Coleman & Anson, 1961; Jaschintski, 1897).

In 4,31 % (McCormack, 1953), the radial artery possesses an unusual course: a dorsal course in the distal third (Otsuka & Terauchi, 1991), a deep course beneath the pronator teres muscle (Small & Millar, 1985) and a superficial course on the brachioradialis muscle (Saski et al., 1999). These variations are explained by the origination of the radial artery from the anterior interosseous artery and the superficial brachial artery, respectively. In those cases a precise examination of the forearm vessels and its dominance is necessary preoperatively. Mc Cormack (1953) described in a study with 750 bodies, the origination of the radial artery from the axillary artery in 2.13%, in 5.7% a superficial brachial artery that courses medial to the biceps muscle, in single cases a superficial radial artery and in 4.43% a median artery. Besides, McCormack found an origination of the ulnar artery from the axillary artery in 0.93%. A median artery originates from the brachial artery and runs through the two bellies of the pronator teres muscle. A superficial ulnar artery is found in about 2-9% (Devansh MS, 1996; McCormack,1953; Weathersby 1956). It runs on the flexor muscles but beneath the palmaris longus muscle and the flexor carpi ulnaris muscle. The last muscle can be absent in these cases. Radial or ulnar artery dominace can be a hint for presence of a superficial ulnar artery or median artery, which can be used for elevation instead of the dominat artery (Bell et al., 2011; Davidson et al., 2009).

The venous drainage of the forearm is guaranteed equally by the subcutaneous veins and the venae commitantes. Consequently, the subcutaneous veins can be preserved or serve for a vein graft. A transplant based on the deep venous system shows advantages in older patients (Weinzweig et al., 1994) and avoids the risk provided by veins venipunctured a few days or weeks ago (Hallock, 1986) and facilitates the prevention of cutaneous nerve damage. The superficial venous system shows high variety in size, dominance and course. Numerous anastomoses exist between the superficial veins, the deep veins and the deep and superficial venous system.

Boutros (2000) described that the lateral antebrachial cutaneous nerve supplies 61.8% of the potential flap area (range 48.3-71.6%), the superficial radial nerve 34.6% (range 26.8-44.1%) and the medial antebrachial cutaneous nerve 33.8% (range 30.5-38.9%).

4. Characteristics

The distinct qualities made the forearm flap to the workhorse in head and neck reconstruction. It is possible to place the flap more proximal or distal without risking the vitality of the flap. The forearm flap provides constant anatomy, is simple and rapid to harvest, possesses many kinds of alternatives in supplying arteries, veins and nerves and shows good vascularisation that results in high vitality and tolerance to radiotherapy (I.A. McGregor & F.M. McGregor, 1986; Soutar & Tanner, 1986). In this regards, this flap excels by its long and large-caliber vascular pedicle and nerves permitting a contralateral anastomosis and the by-passing of vascular defects, even after a neck dissection. The relative large diameter of 2 mm protects from thrombosis and the vessels show seldom sclerotic changes. But de Bree et al. reported a sclerotic impaired radial artery which precluded an anastomosis (DeBree et al., 2004). The flap is thin explaining its pliability, contourability, consistent volume and surface over time. Together with the possibility of harvesting innervated flaps and the relative few hair growth, these are the main reasons for satisfactory aesthetic and intraoral results. Ahcan et al. (2000) described high sensory potency compared to other flaps. The hair growth on the forearm shows some variety, whereas the ulnar side possesses less hair growth in general. To optimize the aesthetic outcome, skin color, texture, hair growth and skin thickness should be evaluated.

The ulnar artery is a little bit shorter than the radial artery. Advantages consist in a less exposed skin area, in a defect that is easier to close, less hair growth and less risk of nerve damage or numb areas. Becker und Gilbert (1988) described a flap based on the dorsal ulnar artery, which originates from the ulnar artery 2-4 cm proximal to the os pisiforme and has a diameter of 0.8-1.2 mm. This variation can be utilised for a fasciocutaneous pedicled flap of 10x5 cm in size, but has a relative short vessel length. The advantages and disadvantages of the forearm flap are summarized in Table 2.

advantages	disadvantages
constant anatomy	discontent of the cosmetic outcome of this exposed area is possible
several altenatives in arteries, veins and nerves	necessity of a preoperative doppler sonography to guarantee the blood supply to the hand
excellent vascularisation: the lenghth of the artery is 10-18 cm, the diameter about 2 mm, almost no sclerotic changes;→important at surgically difficult recipient sites	color differences between the skin of the forearm and the face
flap thickness may be varied by flap placement more distal or proximal	a longer, more pretentious and exhausting operation compared to a local defect closure
simple and rapid to harvest proximal as well as distal	scar tissue fixation between the recipient site and the transplant may occur
thin→no airway obstruction	
pliability, contourability: folding in sandwich technique is possible	
consistent volume and surface over time	
skin with high sensory (protecting) potency	
tolerance to radiation therapy	
infections like osteomyelitis or a osteoradionecrosis often show primary wound healing because of excellent vascularisation	
several skin islands can be raised at the perforators	

Table 2. Advantages and disadvantages of the forearm flap

5. Indications

The forearm serves for a free flap transplant and a pedicled flap as well. Because of the above mentioned advantages and in Table 1 summarized qualtities and characteristics, the forearm flap represents the first therapy option for various kinds of surgical indications with a high overall success rate (Table 3. Complications at the recipient site). It is a highly utilised flap at pretentious recipient sites like the oral cavity, the palate, after a trauma or a tumor resection. The forearm flap replaced the pectoralis major transplant in tongue reconstruction, especially for the oral part of the tongue (Schustermann et al., 1991). The forearm flap particularly serves for the reconstruction of superficial defects. It is used for jaw reconstruction or penile and urethral reconstruction and for coverage of pretibial defects as well, as it is a thin transplant (Biemer, 1988; T.S. Chang and Hwang, 1984). An innervated radial forearm flap is raised with the lateral antebrachial cutaneous nerve and an ulnar forearm flap with the medial antebrachial cutaneous nerve. Innervated flaps could show a faster and increased sensory recovery (Santamaria et al., 1998). Nerve fibers with normal ultrastructure can be found at the recipient site immunohistochemically, in contrast to Waller degeneration and nerve fiber loss in non-innervated flaps (Katou et al., 1995). Boyd et al. (1994) and Dubner et al. (1992) could show that innervated transplants result in an increased sensory capacity of the flap, even improved to the surrounding tissue. The flap should not be raised, if one palmar arch is absent, if there exists an absolute artery dominance or if one forearm artery is missing. Bone should not be included, if it shows osteoporotic changes.

Complications at the recipient site	
Total	10[16 26 41]-39[22 33]
transplant loss	3-13%[7 13 16 25 30 31 33 36 41]
partial transplant loss	1[16 22] -3%[5 17]
thrombosis	2%[16]-9%[22 36]
obstruction of vein grafts	9%[19]
hematoma/seroma	4[21 33]-7%[16 24]
infection	4[16]-12%[33 41]
dehiscence	4[16 41]-12%[33]
fistula formation	pharyngeal: 18-32%[5 15 17 18 29 38 42]/86% close spontaneously[1] oral: 0[5 36]-9%[16 33 35] /83% close spontaneously[1]
stricture, stenosis	8[1 20]-30%[15]
reoperations	3[24]-19%[37]

Table 3. Complications at the recipient site (References are listed under Annexes 9.1 References Table 3)

6. Complications, function loss at the donor site and techniques to minimize

Correct planning and elevation prsupposed, there will be no clinically relevant limitatations in strength, motion and hemodynamics in the forearm and hand after free forearm flap transfer. Sensory and cosmetic outcome is perceived as non-disturbing (Ciuman et al., 2007). The complication rates and the rates of function loss at the donor site are summarized in Table 4.

To optimize the functional and aesthetic outcome at the donor site, different techniques and tests can be applied. A preoperative Doppler sonography is suggested before raising the forearm flap (Dost & Rudofsky, 1993; Dost, 2001). Cases of acute ischemia of the hand were described, although a preoperative assessment with the Allen's test was performed. An absence of a forearm vessel, one palmar arch (in about 4,5%) (Partecke & Buck-Gramcko, 1984), or an absolute dominance of one vessel can lead to an inadequate blood supply of the forearm and hand. Only in those cases, vascular diseases or young patients (Kropfl et al., 1995), a vein graft seems to be profitable (Meland et al., 1993). Heller et al. (2004) described a patient with finger necrosis months after the operation, caused by an absent deep palmar arch, and the subsequent reconstruction of the radial artery. Circia-Llorens et al. (1999) could prove that the remaining forearm vessels, especially the anterior interosseous artery, show an increase in diameter and flow. It could be shown that this vessel forms an anastomosis with the vessel stump of the harvested artery.

Complications at the donor site	
total patients with complications	**14-33%[16 37 41]**
delayed wound healing at the donor site	suprafascial transplant: 0-6-%[2 24] fasciocutaneous transplant: 8-24%[3 16 21 32 37 44]
necrosis above a tendon	3[16]-13%[5 21 32]
hematoma/seroma	2[16]-7%[37]
infection	13%[37]
radius fracture in ostoescutaneous flaps	8-43%[3 7 8 10 32 41 43]
Function loss and long-time results at the donor site	
fasciocutaneous: intact range of wrist motion in 94.4% and free forearm rotation in 97.4%[19] osteocutaneous: intact range of wrist motion in 89-90%[34] after fractures impaired range of motion in up to 50%[3]	
impaired muscle strength	0-16%[11 32 39 40]; after fractures: 50%[3 32]
unsightly scar formation[19]	unstable scar 10.5% level differences 46.8% pigmentation disturbance 58.4% strong plaster over 18.7%
mean circumference loss in fasciocutaneous flaps	1.3%[19]
discontent	2-28%[11 24 27 28 32 41]

Table 4. Frequencies of complications and function loss at the donor site (References are listed under Annexes 9.2 References Table 4)

Wound healing problems can result in impaired functional outcome. A limited wrist and finger motion and decresed muscle strength can result from graft necrosis, exposed tendons, and subsequent adherent scar formation (Kröpfl et al.). A careful coverage of the tendons with flexor muscles guarantees a plain wound for the split-thickness graft. The paratenon should be preserved, the flap can be placed more proximally and the arm should be immobilized in extension to achieve an optimal wound healing. If muscle or bone is included in the flap, the wound healing is delayed and the risk of wound healing problems is increased. Vacuum-technique (Argenta & Morykwas, 1997) can assist wound healing in complicated cases. A short-time hyperalimentation should be considered in tumor patients as well.

A careful preparation, together with an oblique incision to avoid dead space, especially when thick subcutaneous tissue is present, avoid hematoma and seroma formation and leads to an improved healing of the split-thickness graft.

The fracture rate after an osteocutaneous ulnar or radial transplant varies between 8 and 43% but can be decreased by physiotherapy, harvesting not more than one third of the bone, performing a „boat-shaped„ osteotomy, that decreases the stress concentration effect by 5% (Meland et al., 1992), and immobilizing the arm in extension for 6-8 weeks (Partecke & Buck-Gramcko, 1984). A control radiography should be performed before and after the operation.

All different kinds of objective (quantitative, qualitative, dissociated) and subjective sensory impairment were described subsequently to the free forearm flap transfer. But in general, the patient states that he is not affected in his daily activities. Table 5 summarizes the frequencies of disturbed sensory modalities and qualities after free forearm flap transfer.

	Type	Frequency initial	final
quantitative	hypoesthesia, hypopathia, hypoalgesia	16-75% [3,5,9,11,12,21,24,32,41,43]	0[23]- 32%[11,32] 77.1[44]- 86.5%[19] of the defects covered with split-thickness grafts 8,6 % of those areas are anesthetical[44]
	hyperesthesia, hyperalgesia, hyperpathia (neuroma)	5[3]-14%[1,11]	1[19]- 10%[3,11,32] 8.6%[44] of the defects covered with spilt-thickness grafts
qualitative	allesthesia	sporadically, < 3%	only 10[11] -12.4%[19] of the patients have a two-point discrimination on the defects covered with split-thickness grafts
	causalgia/reflex sympathetic dystrophy	sporadically, < 3%	sporadically, < 3%
dissociated	temperature discrimination	cold intolerance with improvement with time 0-32%[1,3,6,7,11,12,14,24,32,43,44] (climate dependency) single cases of heat intolerance[39]	
subjective	itching	initially manifesting subjective sensory dysfunction often signals nerve regeneration or nerve ingrowth	14[12]- 19.6%[11,19]
	dysesthesia hypersensitiveness		10[11]-40.6%[19] 29.5%, but in only 1,1% pronounced[19]
	scar pain		3[11]-36%; 6.5% of them are distinct or strong[19]

Table 5. Frequencies of sensory impairment at the donor site after fasciocutaneous forarm flap transfer (References are listed under Annexes 9.3 References Table 5)

Initially, sensory disturbances can be found in 17-75% but decrease during the next months. Hypersensitiveness, paresthesias and dysesthesias can signal sensory regeneration. However, hyperesthesia and neuralgia could signal nerve section, but decrease in the following months, too. Together with pain due to neuroma formation or causalgia, they are difficult to treat, what underlines the importance of careful preparation and good vascularisation to prevent perineural scar formation and assist nerve regeneration. Richardson et al. (1997) described four neuromas in a group of 86 patients making a surgical neuroma excision necessary (Anthony et al., 1994). The nerve endings should be covered with muscle and not come into contact with the split-thickness skin graft. Although it is not possible to preserve the cutaneous nerves in each case, e.g. the lateral antebrachial cutaneous nerve or the superficial radial nerve, an ulnar-based flap and the limitated dimension to the radial or ulnar border can improve sensory outcome (Lovie et al., 1984).

It is not surprising that women are more pretentious with regard to the aesthetic outcome at the forearm. Alternatives for achieving the optimal cosmetic result are dicussed in Table 1 and the following paragraph. Hülsbergen-Krüger et al. (1996) described in their group of 267 patients after closing the defect with split-thickness graft, reduced pigmentation in 43.4%, increased pigmentation in 15%, level differences > 0.1 cm in 46.8%, but in only 12% >0.4 cm, an unstable scar in 10.5% and an adherence of the defect in 18.7%. Adequate compression, first with dressings and later with compression stockings, and the application of 2 mm metal plates can assist the wound healing.

7. Closure of the donor site

The most utilised technique to close the defect at the donor site is the coverage with 0.2-0.6 mm split-thickness skin grafts. Lutz and colleagues described a success rate of 98% compared with 84% in full skin grafts (Lutz et al., 1999). However, if the wound is not plain, e.g. above a tendon, opposite results can be found as well. Other studies showed a complete loss of the split-thickness skin graft in 8 (Evans et al., 1994) -16% (Richardson et al., 1997), a partial loss in 16-35% (Bardsley et al., 1990; A.D. McGregor, 1987; Meland et al., 1993, Richardson et al., 1997; Swanson et al., 1990; Timmons et al., 1986), and a loss of split-thickness skin grafts in suprafascial elevated flaps in 0-4% (Avery et al., 2001, Chang et al., 1996, Lutz et al., 1999). Patients are more content with full skin grafts than with split-thickness grafts: 92% to 57% (Lutz et al., 1999). Defects up to 4x8 cm in size can be closed with a V-Y transposition flap (Elliot et al., 1996). Enough skin should be disposable to avoid limitations in wrist extension, chronic lymphatic edema, sensory disturbance of the forearm or necrosis. Another alternative of closure is skin expansion that can be primary (Bardsley et al., 1990; Herndl & Mühlbauer, 1986) or secondary. Because of wound healing problems in about 30%, Hallock (1988) recommends for the secondary skin expansion a coverage with split-thickness skin graft , in the first instance. After six weeks, it is possible to begin the expansion. A secondary shrinking and a thinning out of the subcutaneous tissue needs to be considered. The skin area of the harvested transplant should never be expanded as a shrinking at the recipient site would be the consequence. The flap preparation should begin from the region opposite to the expanded area to avoid shrinking during the operation. However, a disturbance of the microcirculation with venous congestion might still occur. Dehiscence after expansion was described in up to 40% (Bootz et al., 1993; Lovie et al., 1984), but other studies showed complication rates of less than 10% (Makitie et al., 1997).

8. Conclusion

Microvascular surgery often presents the only possibility to reach satisfactory functional, and cosmetic outcomes and to achieve acceptable quality of life for reconstruction in the head and neck. Due to distinct charactersitics the forearm flap is one of the most used transplants for reconstruction in the head and neck and a widely used transplant for other indications as well. Correct planning and elevation presupposed the flap success rates average at least 90% with no relevant limitations in strength, motion and hemodynamics in the forearm or hand and non-disturbing sensory and cosmetic outcome at the donor site.

9. Annexes

9.1 References Table 3

Complications at the recipient site

9.2 References Table 4

Frequencies of complications and function loss at the donor site

9.3 References Table 5

Frequencies of sensory impairment at the donor site after fasciocutaneous forarm flap transfer

[1] Anthony JP, Singer MI, Deschler DG. Dougherty ET, Reed CG & Kaplan MJ. (1994). Long-term functional results after pharyngoesophageal reconstruction with the radial forearm free flap. *Am J Surg,* 168(5), pp. 441-445. ISSN: 0002-9610

[2] Avery CM, Pereira J & Brown AE. (2001). Suprafascial dissection of the radial forearm flap and donor site morbidity. *Int J Oral Maxillofac Surg,* 30(1), pp. 42-48. ISSN: 0901-5027

[3] Bardsley AF, Soutar DS, Elliot D & Batchelor AG. (1990). Reducing morbidity in the radial forearm flap donor site. *Plast Reconstr Surg,* 86(2), pp. 287-294. ISSN: 0032-1052

[4] Becker C & Gilbert A. (1988) The ulnar flap. (German). *Handchir Mikrochir Plast Chir,* 20(4), pp. 180-183. ISSN: 0722-1819

[5] Blackwell KE. (1999). Unsurpassed reliability of free flaps for head and neck reconstruction. *Arch Otolaryngol Head Neck Surg,* 125(3), pp. 295-299. ISSN: 0886-4470

[6] Bootz F, Becker D & Fliesek J. (1993). Functional results and survival of tumor patients after reconstruction of the mouth cavity and oropharynx using a microvascular radial forearm flap. (German). *HNO,* 41(8), pp. 542-552. ISSN: 0017-6192

[7] Boorman JG, Brown JA & Sykes PJ. (1987). Morbidity in the forearm flap donor arm. *Br J Plast Surg,* 40(2), pp. 207-212. ISSN: 0007-1226

[8] Boyd JB, Rosen I, Rotstein L, Freeman J, Gullane P, Manktelow R & Zuker R. (1990). The iliac crest and the radial forearm flap in vascularized oromandibular reconstruction. *Am J Surg,* 159(3), pp. 301-308. ISSN:0002-9610

[9] Brown MT, Couch E & Huchton DM. (1999). Assessment of donor-site function morbidity from radial forearm fasciocutaneous free flap harvest. *Arch Otolaryngol Head Neck Surg,* 125(12), pp. 1371-1374. ISSN: 0886-4470

[10] Christie DR, Duncan GM & Glasson DW. (1994). The ulnar artery free flap: the first 7 years. *Plast Reconstr Surg,* 93(3), pp. 547-551. ISSN: 0032-1052

[11] Ciuman R, Mohr C, Kröger K & Dost P. (2007). The forearm flap: assessment of functional and aesthetic outcomes and quality of life. *Am J of Otolaryngol,* 28(6), pp. 367-374. ISSN: 0196-0709

[12] DeBree R, Hartley C, Smeele LE, Kuik DJ, Quak JJ & Leemans CR. (2004). Evaluation of Donor Site Function and Morbidity of the fasciocutaneous radial forearm flap. *Laryngoscope,* 114(11), pp. 1973-1976. ISSN: 1531-4995

[13] Dost P. (2001). The ulnar artery or the radial artery can be used alternatively in the free underarm flap. (German). *Laryngorhinootologie,* 80(3), pp. 152-155. ISSN: 0935-8943

[14] Dost P. & Rudofsky G. (1993). Doppler ultrasonography as a pre-operative aid to base the forearm flap on the radial or ulnar artery. *Clin Otolaryngol Allied Sci,* 18(5), pp. 355-358. ISSN: 1749-4478

[15] Endo T & Nakayama Y. (1997). Pharyngoesophageal reconstruction: a clinical comparison between free tensor fasciae latae and radial forearm flaps. *J Reconstr Microsurg,* 13(2), pp. 93-97. ISSN: 0743-684X

[16] Evans GR, Schustermann MA, Kroll SS, Miller MJ, Reece GP, Robb GL, Ainslie N. (1994). The radial forearm free flap for head and neck reconstruction: a review. *Am J Surg,* 168(5), pp. 446-450. ISSN: 0002-9610

[17] Hagen R. (1991). Stimmrehabilitation mit dem Unterarmlappen. (German). In: *Konturen der plastischen Chirurgie,* Greulich M, Wangerin K, Gubisch W, eds. pp. 55-62, Hans Marseille Verlag, ISBN: 3886160440, München

[18] Harii K, Ebihara S, Ono I, Saito H, Terui S & Takato T. (1985). Pharyngoesophageal reconstruction using a fabricated forearm free flap. *Plast Reconstr Surg,* 75(4), pp. 463-476. ISSN: 0032-1052

[19] Hülsbergen-Krüger S, Müller K & Partecke BD. (1996). Donor site defect after removal of free and pedicled forearm flaps: functional and cosmetic results. (German). *Handchir Mikrochir Plast Chir,* 28, 82(2), pp. 70-75. ISSN: 0722-1819

[20] Kelly KE, Anthony JP & Singer M. (1994). Pharyngoesophageal reconstruction using the radial forearm fasciocutaneous free flap: Preliminary results. *Otolaryngol Head Neck Surg,* 111(1), pp. 16-24. ISSN: 0194-5998

[21] Kröpfl A, Helmberger R, Gasperschlitz F, Moosmüller W & Hertz H. (1995). Donor site morbidity following radial forearm flap.(German). *Handchir Mikrochir Plast Chir,* 27(2), pp. 72-77. ISSN: 0722-1819

[22] Kroll SS, Schustermann MA, Reece GP, Miller MJ, Evans GR, Robb GL & Baldwin BJ. (1996). Choice of flap and incidence of free flap success. *Plast Reconstr Surg,* 98(3), pp. 459-463. ISSN: 0032-1052

[23] Lovie MJ, Duncan GM & Glasson DW. (1984). The ulnar artery forearm flap. *Br J Plast Surg,* 37(4), pp. 486-492. ISSN: 0007-1226

[24] Lutz BS, Chang SCN, Chuang SS & Wei FC. (1999). Supra-fascial elevated free forearm flap-indications, surgical technique and follow-up examination of the donor site defect. (German). *Handchir Mikrochir Plast Chir,* 31(1), pp. 10-14, ISSN: 0722-1819

[25] Makitie A, Aitasalo K, Pukander J, VirtaniemiJ, Hyrynkangas K, et al. (1997). Microvascular free flaps in head and neck cancer surgery in Finland 1986-1995. *Acta Otolaryngol Suppl,* 529, pp. 245-246. ISSN: 0365-5237

[26] Matthew WR & Hochman M. (2000). Length of stay after free flap reconstruction of the head and neck. *Laryngoscope,* 110(2), pp. 210-216. ISSN: 1531-4995

[27] McGregor AD. (1987). The free radial forearm flap: The management of the secondary defect. *Br J Plast Surg,* 40(1), pp. 83. ISSN: 0007-1226

[28] Meland BN, Core GB & Hoverman VR. (1993). The radial forearm flap donor site: Should we vein graft the artery? A comparative study. *Plast Reconstr Surg,* 91(5), pp. 865-870. ISSN: 0032-1052

[29] Percival NJ & Early MJ. (1989). Pharyngostome closure using the radial forearm free flap. *Br J Plast Surg,* 42(4), pp. 473-477. ISSN: 0007-1226

[30] Plinkert PK, Bootz F & Zenner HP. Differential indications of free and pedicled transplants in reconstructive surgery in the head and neck area. (1993).(German). *Laryngorhinootologie,* 72(11), pp. 537-544. ISSN: 0935-8943

[31] Remmert S. (1995). Microvascular anastomoses in reconstructive head and neck surgery. (German). *Laryngorhinootologie,* 74(4), pp. 233-237. ISSN: 0935-8943

[32] Richardson D, Fisher, SE, Vaughan, ED & Brown JS. (1997). Radial forearm flap donor-site complications and morbidity: A prospective study. *Plast Reconstr Surg,* 99(1), pp. 109-115. ISSN: 0032-1052

[33] Schustermann MA, Kroll SS, Weber RS, Byers RM, Guillamondegqui O & Goepfert H. (1991). Intraoral soft tissue reconstruction after cancer ablation: A comparison of the pectoralis major flap and the free radial forearm flap. *Am J Surg,* 162(4), pp. 397-399. ISSN: 0002-9610

[34] Smith AA, Bowen CV, Rabaczak T & Boyd JB. (1994). Donor site deficit of the osteocutaneous radial forearm flap. *Ann Plast Surg,* 32(4), pp. 372-376. ISSN: 0148-7043

[35] Soutar DS. (1989). Radial forearm flaps. In: *Microsurgical reconstruction of the head and neck,* Baker SR, editor. pp. 64-76. Churchill Livingstone, ISBN: 0443085870, New York

[36] Soutar DS & McGregor IA. (1986). The radial forearm flap in intraoral reconstruction: The experience of 60 consecutive cases. *Plast Reconstr Surg,* 78(1), pp. 1-8. ISSN: 0032-1052

[37] Stark B, Nathanson A, Heden P & Jernbeck J. (1998). Results after resection of intraoral cancer and reconstruction with the free radial forearm flap. *ORL J Otorhinolaryngol Relat Spec ,* 60(4), pp. 212-217. ISSN: 0301-1569.

[38] Su WF, Chen SG & Sheng H. (2002). Speech and swallowing function after reconstruction with a redial forearm free flap or a pectoralis major flap for tongue cancer. *J Formos Med Assoc,* 101(7), pp. 472-477. ISSN: 0929-6646

[39] Suominen S & Asko-Seljavaara S. (1996). Thermography of hands after a radial forearm flap has been raised. *Scand J Plast. Reconstr Hand Surg,* 30(4), pp. 307-314. ISSN: 0284-4311

[40] Suominen S, Ahovuo J & Asko-Seljavaara S. (1996). Donor site morbidity of radial forearm flaps. *Scand J Plast. Reconstr Hand Surg,* 30(1), pp. 57-61. ISSN: 0284-4311

[41] Swanson E, Boyd JB & Manktelow RT. (1990). The radial forearm flap: Reconstructive applications and donor-site defects in 35 consecutive patients. *Plast Reconstr Surg,* 85(2), pp. 258-266. ISSN: 0032-1052

[42] Takato T, Harii K, Ebihara S, Ono I, Yoshizumi T & Nakatsuka T. (1987). Oral and pharyngeal reconstruction using the free forearm flap. *Arch Otolaryngol Head Neck Surg,* 113(8), pp. 873-879. ISSN: 0886-4470

[43] Timmons MJ, Missotten FEM, Poole MD & Davies DM. (1986). Complications of radial forearm flap donor sites. *Br J Plast Surg,* 39(2), pp. 176-178. ISSN: 0007-1226

[44] Toschka H, Feifel H, Erli, HJ, Minkenberg R, Paar O & Riediger D. (2001). Aesthetic and functional results of harvesting radial forearm flap, especially with regard to hand function. *Int J Oral Maxillofac Surg,* 30(1), pp. 42-48. ISSN: 0901-5027

10. References

Ahcan U, Arnez Z & Kristian A. (2000). Physiological differences for distinct somatic sensory modalities and sweating among the donor sites of cutaneous and fasciocutaneous free flaps. *Acta Chir Plast,* 42(1), pp. 7-12. ISSN:0001-5423

Anthony JP, Singer MI, Deschler DG. Dougherty ET, Reed CG & Kaplan MJ. (1994). Long-term functional results after pharyngoesophageal reconstruction with the radial forearm free flap. *Am J Surg,* 168(5), pp. 441-445. ISSN: 0002-9610

Argenta LC & Morykwas MJ. (1997). Vacuum-assisted closure: a new method for wound control and treatment: clinical experience. *Ann Plast Surg,* 38(6), pp. 563-576. ISSN: 0148-7043

Avery CM, Pereira J & Brown AE. (2001). Suprafascial dissection of the radial forearm flap and donor site morbidity. *Int J Oral Maxillofac Surg,* 30(1), pp. 42-48. ISSN: 0901-5027

Bardsley AF, Soutar DS, Elliot D & Batchelor AG. (1990). Reducing morbidity in the radial forearm flap donor site. *Plast Reconstr Surg,* 86(2), pp. 287-294. ISSN: 0032-1052

Becker C & Gilbert A. (1988) The ulnar flap. (German). *Handchir Mikrochir Plast Chir,* 20(4), pp. 180-183. ISSN: 0722-1819

Bell RA, Schneider DS & Wax MK. (2011). Superficial ulnar artery: a contraindication to radial forearm free tissue transfer. *Laryngoscope,* 121(5), pp. 933-936, ISSN: 1531-4995

Biemer E. (1988). Penile construction by the radial arm flap. *Clin Plast Surg,* 15(3), pp. 425-430. ISSN: 0094-1298

Biemer E & Stock W. (1983). Total thumb reconstruction: A one-stage reconstruction using an osteocutaneous forearm flap. *Br J Plast Surg,* 36(1), pp. 52-55. ISSN: 0007-1226

Bootz F, Becker D & Fliesek J. (1993). Functional results and survival of tumor patients after reconstruction of the mouth cavity and oropharynx using a microvascular radial forearm flap. (German). *HNO,* 41(8), pp. 542-552. ISSN: 0017-6192

Boutros S, Yuksel E, Weinfeld AB, Alford EL & Netscher DT. (2000). Neural anatomy of the radial forearm flap. *Ann Plast Surg,* 44(4), pp. 375-380. ISSN: 0148-7043

Boyd B, Mulholand S, Gullane P, Irish J, Kelly L, Rotstein L & Brown D. (1994). Reinnervated lateral antebrachial cutaneous neurosome flaps in oral reconstruction. *Plast Reconstr Surg,* 93(7), pp. 1350-1362. ISSN: 0032-1052

Cavanagh S, Pho, RW & Kour AK. (1991). A composite neuro-teno-cutaneous forearm flap in the one-stage reconstruction of a large defect of the soft tissue around the ankle. *J Reconstr Microsurg,* 7(4), pp. 323-329. ISSN: 0743-684X

Chang SC, Miller, G, Halbert CF, Yang KH, Chao WC & Wei FC. (1996). Limiting donor site morbidity by suprafascial dissection of the radial forearm flap. *Microsurgery,* 17(3), pp. 136-140. ISSN: 1098-2752.

Chang TS & Hwang WY. (1984). Forearm flap in one-stage reconstruction of the penis. *Plast Reconstr Surg,* 74(2), pp. 251-258. ISSN: 0032-1052

Circia-Llorens G, Gomez-Cia T & Talegon-Melendez A. (1999). Analysis of flow changes in forearm arteries after raising the radial forearm flap: a prospective study using colour duplex imaging. *Plast Reconstr Surg,* 52(2), pp. 440-44. ISSN: 0032-1052

Ciuman R, Mohr C, Kröger K & Dost P. (2007). The forearm flap: assessment of functional and aesthetic outcomes and quality of life. *Am J of Otolaryngol,* 28(6), pp. 367-374. ISSN: 0196-0709

Coleman SS & Anson BJ. (1961). Arterial patterns in the hand based upon a study of 650 specimen. *Surg Gynec Obstet,* 113, pp. 409-424. ISSN: 0039-6087

Costa H, Cunha C, Guimaraes I, Comba S, Malta A & Lopes A. (1993). Prefabricated flaps for the head and neck: a preliminary report. *Br J Plast Surg,* 46(3), pp. 223-227. ISSN: 0007-1226

Davidson JS & Pichora DR. (2009). Median artery flap. *Ann Plast Surg,* 62(6), pp. 627-629. ISSN: 0148-7043

DeBree R, Quak JJ, Kummer JA, Simsek S & Leemans CR. (2004). Severe atherosclerosis of the radial artery in a free radial forearm flap precluding its use. *Oral Oncol,* 40(1), pp. 99-102. ISSN: 1368-8375

Devansh MS. (1996). Superficial ulnar artery flap. *Plast Reconstr Surg,* 97(2), pp. 420-426. ISSN: 0032-1052

Dost P. (2001). The ulnar artery or the radial artery can be used alternatively in the free underarm flap. (German). *Laryngorhinootologie,* 80(3), pp. 152-155. ISSN: 0935-8943

Dost P. & Rudofsky G. (1993). Doppler ultrasonography as a pre-operative aid to base the forearm flap on the radial or ulnar artery. *Clin Otolaryngol Allied Sci,* 18(5), pp. 355-358. ISSN: 1749-4478

Dubner S & Heller KS. (1992). Reinnervated radial forearm free flaps in head and neck reconstruction. *J Reconstr Microsurg,* 8(6), pp. 467-470. ISSN: 0743-684X

Elliot D, Bardsley AF, Batchelor AG &Soutar DS. (1996). Direct closure of the radial forearm flap donor defect. *Br J Plast Surg,* 41(4), pp. 354-357. ISSN: 0007-1226

Evans GR, Schustermann MA, Kroll SS, Miller MJ, Reece GP, Robb GL, Ainslie N. (1994). The radial forearm free flap for head and neck reconstruction: a review. *Am J Surg,* 168(5), pp. 446-450. ISSN: 0002-9610

Hallock GG. (1986). Caution in using the Chinese radial forearm flap. *Plast Reconstr Surg,* 77, pp. 164. ISSN: 0032-1052

Hallock GG. (1988). Refinement of the radial forearm flap donor site using skin expansion. *Plast Reconstr Surg,* 81(1), pp. 21-25. ISSN: 0032-1052

Hashikawa K, Tahara S, Ishida H, Yokoo S, Sanno T, Terashi H & Nibu K. (2006). Simple reconstruction with titanium mesh and radial forearm flap after globe-sparing total maxillectomy: a 5-year follow-up study. *Plast Reconstr Surg,* 117(3), pp. 963-967. ISSN: 0032-1052

Heller F, Wei W & Wei, FC. (2004). Chronic arterial insufficiency of the hand with fingertip necrosis 1 year after harvesting a radial forearm free flap. *Plast Reconstr Surg,* 114(3), pp. 728-731. ISSN: 0032-1052

Herndl E & Mühlbauer W. (1986). Direct closure of donor defects of the radial flap by preliminary stretching of the skin with a skin expander. (German). *Handchir Mikrochir Plast Chir,* 18(5), pp. 289-290. ISSN: 0722-1819

Hülsbergen-Krüger S, Müller K & Partecke BD. (1996). Donor site defect after removal of free and pedicled forearm flaps: functional and cosmetic results. (German). *Handchir Mikrochir Plast Chir,* 28, 82(2), pp. 70-75. ISSN: 0722-1819

Jaschintski SN. 1897. Morphologie und Topographie des Arcus volaris sublimus und profundus des Menschen. (German). *Anat Hefte,* 7:163-188. ISSN: 0177-5154

Katou F, Shirai N, Kamakura S, Ohki H, Motegi K, Andoh N, Date F & Nagura H. (1995). Intraoral reconstruction with innervated radial forearm flap. *Oral Surg Oral Med Oral Pathol,* 80(6), pp. 638-644. ISSN: 1079-2104

Kröpfl A, Helmberger R, Gasperschlitz F, Moosmüller W & Hertz H. (1995). Donor site morbidity following radial forearm flap.(German). *Handchir Mikrochir Plast Chir,* 27(2), pp. 72-77. ISSN: 0722-1819

Kubo T, Tomita K, Takada A, Yano K & Hosokawa K. (2009). Reconstruction of adult auricular defect with thin titanium mesh and prelaminated free radial forearm flap. *Scand J Plast Reconstr Surg Hand Surg,* 43(1), pp. 54-57. ISSN: 0284-4311

Lovie MJ, Duncan GM & Glasson DW. (1984). The ulnar artery forearm flap. *Br J Plast Surg,* 37(4), pp. 486-492. ISSN: 0007-1226

Lutz BS, Chang SCN, Chuang SS & Wei FC. (1999). Supra-fascial elevated free forearm flap-indications, surgical technique and follow-up examination of the donor site defect. (German). *Handchir Mikrochir Plast Chir,* 31(1), pp. 10-14, ISSN: 0722-1819

Makitie A, Aitasalo K, Pukander J, VirtaniemiJ, Hyrynkangas K, et al. (1997). Microvascular free flaps in head and neck cancer surgery in Finland 1986-1995. *Acta Otolaryngol Suppl,* 529, pp. 245-246. ISSN: 0365-5237

McGregor AD. (1987). The free radial forearm flap: The management of the secondary defect. *Br J Plast Surg,* 40(1), pp. 83. ISSN: 0007-1226

McGregor IA & McGregor FM. (1986). *Cancer of the face and mouth: Pathology and Management for Surgeons.* pp.51-53, Churchill Livingstone, ISBN: 0443024553, Edinburgh

McCormack L, Cauldwell EW & Anson BJ. (1953). Brachial and antebrachial arterial patterns. *Surg Gynec Obstet,* 96(1), pp. 43-54. ISSN: 0039-6087.

Meland NB, Maki S, Chao EY & Rademaker B. (1992). The radial forearm flap: A biomechanical study of donor-site morbidity utilizing sheep tibia. *Plast Reconstr Surg,* 90(5), pp. 763-773. ISSN: 0032-1052

Meland BN, Core GB & Hoverman VR. (1993). The radial forearm flap donor site: Should we vein graft the artery? A comparative study. *Plast Reconstr Surg,* 91(5), pp. 865-870. ISSN: 0032-1052

Mühlbauer W, Herndl E & Stock W. (1982). The forearm flap. *Plast Reconstr Surg,* 70(3), pp. 336-342. ISSN: 0032-1052

Otsuka T & Terauchi M. (1991). An anomaly of the radial artery-relevance for the forearm flap. *Br J Plast Surg,* 44(5), pp. 390-391. ISSN: 0007-1226

Partecke BD & Buck-Gramcko D. (1984). Free forearm flap for reconstruction of soft tissue defect concurrent with improved peripheral circulation. *J Reconstr Microchir,* 1(1), pp. 1-6. ISSN: 0743-684X

Partecke BD, Buck-Gramcko D & Pachnucki A. (1986). Use of a fascia flap of the forearm in soft tissue defects of the extremities. (German). *Handchir Mikrochir Plast Chir,* 18(6), pp. 353-355. ISSN: 0722-1819

Pribaz JJ & Fine NA. (1994). Prelamination: defining the prefabricated flap-a case report and review. *Microsurgery,* 15(9), pp. 618-623. ISSN: 1098-2752

Rath T, Millesi W, Millesi-Schobel G, Lang S, Glaser C & Todoroff B. (1997). Mucosal prelaminated flaps for physiological reconstruction of intraoral defects after resection. *Br J Plast Surg,* 50(5), 303-307. ISSN: 0007-1226

Richardson D, Fisher, SE, Vaughan, ED & Brown JS. (1997). Radial forearm flap donor-site complications and morbidity: A prospective study. *Plast Reconstr Surg,* 99(1), pp. 109-115. ISSN: 0032-1052

Santamaria E, Wei FC, Chen IH & Chuang DC. (1998). Sensation recovery on innervated radial forearm flap for hemiglossectomy reconstruction by using different recipient nerves. *Plast Reconstr Surg,* 103(2), pp. 450-457. ISSN: 0032-1052

Saski K, Nozaki M, Aiba H, & Isono N. (1999). A rare variant of the radial artery: clinical considerations in raising a radial forearm flap. *Br J Plast Surg,* 53(5), pp. 445-447. ISSN: 0007-1226

Schustermann MA, Kroll SS, Weber RS, Byers RM, Guillamondegqui O & Goepfert H. (1991). Intraoral soft tissue reconstruction after cancer ablation: A comparison of the pectoralis major flap and the free radial forearm flap. *Am J Surg,* 162(4), pp. 397-399. ISSN: 0002-9610

Small JO & Millar R. (1985). The radial forearm flap: an anomaly of the radial artery. *Br J Plast Surg,* 38(4), pp. 501. ISSN: 0007-1226

Soutar DS & McGregor IA. (1986). The radial forearm flap in intraoral reconstruction: The experience of 60 consecutive cases. *Plast Reconstr Surg,* 78(1), pp. 1-8. ISSN: 0032-1052

Soutar DS & Tanner NSB. (1986). The radial forearm flap in managing soft tissue injuries of the hand. *Br J Plast Surg,* 37(1), pp. 18-26. ISSN: 0007-1226

Stock W, Mühlbauer W & Biemer E. (1981). The neurovascular forearm island flap. (German). *Z Plast Chir,* 5(3), pp. 158-165. ISSN: 0342-7978

Swanson E, Boyd JB & Manktelow RT. (1990). The radial forearm flap: Reconstructive applications and donor-site defects in 35 consecutive patients. *Plast Reconstr Surg,* 85(2), pp. 258-266. ISSN: 0032-1052

Timmons MJ, Missotten FEM, Poole MD & Davies DM. (1986). Complications of radial forearm flap donor sites. *Br J Plast Surg,* 39(2), pp. 176-178. ISSN: 0007-1226

Weathersby HT. (1956). Unusual variation of the ulnar artery. *Anat Rec,* 124(2), pp. 245-248. ISSN: 0003-276X

Webster HR & Robinson DW. (1995). The radial forearm flap without fascia and other refinements. *Eur J Plast Surg,* 18, pp. 11-13. ISSN: 0930-343X

Weinzweig N, Chen L & Chen ZW. (1994). The distally based radial forearm fasciocutaneous flap with preservation of the radial artery: An anatomic and clinical approach. *Plast Reconstr Surg,* 94(5), pp. 675-684. ISSN: 0032-1052

Wolff KD, Ervens J & Hoffmeister B. (1995). Improvement of the radial forearm donor site by prefabrication of fascial-split-thickness skin grafts. *Plast Reconstr Surg,* 98(2), pp. 358-361. ISSN: 0032-1052

Yang G, Chen B, Gao Y, Liu X, Li J, Jiang S & He S. (1981). Forearm free skin flap transplantation. *Natl Med J China,* 61:139-141. ISSN: 0376-2491.

4

Mandibular Condylar Hiperplasia

Everton Da Rosa, Júlio Evangelista De Souza Júnior and
Melina Spinosa Tiussi
Hospital de Base do Distrito Federal
Brazil

1. Introduction

1.1 Asymmetry

The term symmetry was defined as the mathematical identity between the mirror images of the right and left halves of an object. However, it is rare for humans to have such mathematical symmetry in the craniofacial skeleton[1]. Robinson et al reported that a beautiful face should be harmonious with comparable size and position of the skeletal structures and soft tissues[2]. They stated that a favorable face can be shown by the soft tissues[2]. For patients with maxillofacial deformity, facial asymmetry is a common chief complaint, although patients might have other sagittal or vertical jaw imbalances concomitantly[1]. In contrast, facial asymmetry might be masked by severe facial skeletal imbalance, dental malalignment, soft tissue compensation, or tilting of head posture[1]. The documented prevalence of facial asymmetry ranges from 21% to 85%[1]. Usually the structures of the lower face are more asymmetric than those of the upper face[1].

Bishara et al, 1994, in a review of dental and facial asymmetries, showed that many factors are implicated in asymmetry: genetic or congenital malformations such as hemifacial microsomia, environmental factors such as habits and trauma, functional deviations, and so on[3]. Asymmetry can have different characteristics even with the same etiology because it can be influenced by other factors such as onset, individual growth, and compensation[3].

Although the nature of asymmetry is complex and its characteristics are diverse, approaches to systematic classification of facial asymmetry have been few[4]. Hinds et al, 1960, classified mandibular asymmetry into 2 categories: unilateral condylar hyperplasia and deviation prognathism[5]. Rowe, 1960 classified asymmetry into 3 groups: unilateral condylar hyperplasia, unilateral macrognathia confined to the skeletal element only, and unilateral macrognathia of both osseous and muscular components[6]. Bruce and Hayward, in 1968, classified mandibular asymmetry into deviation prognathism, unilateral condylar hyperplasia and unilateral macrognathia[7]. Obwegeser, 1986, suggested classifying asymmetries as either a hemimandibular elongation or a hemimandibular hyperplasia[8]. Bishara et al, 1994, classified dentofacial asymmetry into dental, skeletal, muscular, and functional[3].

Asymmetries can be assessed by clinical evaluation, photographs, posteroanterior (PA) cephalograms and 3D computed tomography (CT) scans. On physical examination, asymmetries becomes most apparent when the patient smiles[9]. At rest, however, the presence of an elevated labial commissure or alar base on one side is often an indication of vertical skeletal asymmetry[9]. This should be documented during routine evaluation of patients for orthodontic or orthognathic surgical treatment. To measure occlusal canting, a wooden tongue depressor can be placed across the right and left posterior teeth, and the parallelism or the angle of the tongue depressor to the interpupillary plane can be documented[9]. Alternatively, the vertical distance between the maxillary canines and the medial canthi of the eyes can be measured[9].

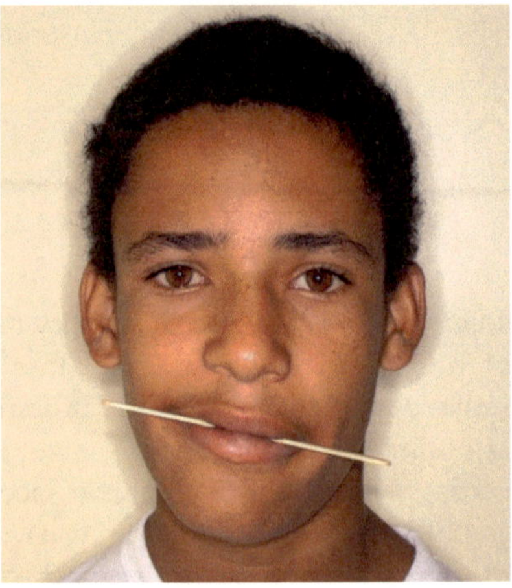

Fig. 1. Measuring occlusal canting

Other important tools for objective evaluation of face symmetry are photographs. Ferrario et al used digitized photographic analysis to determine angulation of the occlusal plane[1]. A mean angulation from 2.15° to 2.90° was found in healthy normal patients[1]. For evaluation of skeletal and dental structures, posteroanterior (PA) cephalogram is commonly used as an effective tool to quantify asymmetry. By identifying the horizontal and midsagittal reference planes, the difference in the distance of the counterpart land-marks on each half of the skeleton can be measured and calculated[1]. Analysis of the PA cephalogram also can be used to determine occlusal cant[9]. A line is drawn connecting the occlusal surfaces of the left and right maxillary first molars. The angle of this plane relative to the transverse axis of the skull, that is, the angle of occlusal cant, is measured[9].

On last decades, 3D computed tomography (CT) scans has helped surgeons to improve evaluation, planning and accuracy of orthognathic surgery. With this new technology, it is possible to create 3D models of the face that incorporate accurate renditions of the teeth, skeleton, and soft tissues. These techniques are more important in the assessment of asymmetries, since in PA cephalograms all facial structures are projected onto a single sagittal plane[10].

The decision of surgical correction of facial asymmetry might depend on patients awareness of the esthetic problem, extent of occlusal deterioration, and concomitant sagittal or vertical jaw imbalance[1]. It has been suggested that a level occlusal plane is a prerequisite for success in all orthognathic surgeries[1]. Two-jaw orthognathic surgery might be necessary in cases with obvious cant of the frontal occlusal plane[1]. Treatment goals of orthognathic correction in facial asymmetry should consist of correlated maxillary midline to facial midline, level oral commissures, symmetric appearance of bilateral maxillary canines and correlated chin point to facial midline. Ideally the planned surgical prediction of the frontal occlusal plane should be parallel to the orbital plane on PA cephalograms; the central contact of maxillary inci-sors and chin point (menton) should be in the mid-sagittal plane; and the axis of the front teeth should parallel the midsagittal plane[1].

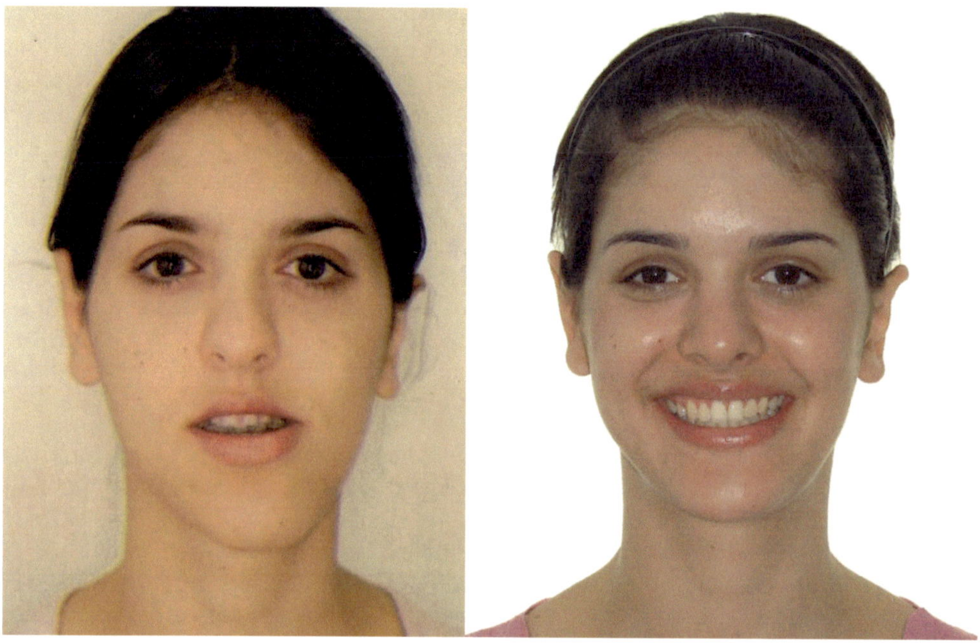

Fig. 2. Face balance after orthognathic surgery with high condylectomy in treatment of condylar hiperplasia

2. Mandibular condylar hyperplasia (CH)

Mandibular condylar hyperplasia (CH) is a non-neoplasic rare malformation that changes morphology and size of mandibular condyles[11]. It was first described by Robert Adams in 1836 as a condition that causes overdevelopment of the mandible, creating functional and esthetic problems[12]. The excessive unilateral growth of the mandibular condyle can lead to facial asymmetry, occlusal disturbance, and joint dysfunction[13]. It represents a challenge to both surgeons and orthodontists and because of the severe dentofacial deformity it can create[14]. A complete understanding of the nature of the deformity, etiology, clinical presentation, options for treatment, and timing of treatment is required in order to achieve optimal treatment outcomes[14].

2.1 Etiology and diagnosis

The etiology of condylar hyperplasia is controversial and not well understood[15]. CH usually develops during puberty and rarely begins after the age of 20[14]. The identification of sex hormone receptors in and around the temporomandibular joint (TMJ) and the pubertal onset of CH strongly suggest a hormonal influence in the etiology[14]. Suggested theories include trauma followed by excessive proliferation in repair, infection, hormonal influences, arthrosis, hypervascularity, and a possible ge-netic role[16]. Obwegeser and Makek suggested that different growth factors individually controlling generalized hypertrophy and elongation might be responsible for the deformities[8]. Another possible cause being taken into consideration, but thus far not substantiated, is an increase in functional loading of the TMJ[16].

CH occurs with equal frequency in males and females, as well as unilaterally and bilaterally[14]. These patients usually demonstrate a Class I or mild Class III skeletal and occlusal relationship before the onset of CH and develop into a Class III or severe Class III relationship as their growth accelerates[14]. CH usually begins during the second decade of life around the pubertal growth phase and can continue into the middle or late 20s[14]. The condyles growth pattern, in terms of magnitude, rate, and direction, can influence the timing of surgery and the types of corrective surgical procedures necessary[14]. Ninety-eight percent of facial growth is completed by age 15 in females and by age 17 or 18 in males[19]. During the pubertal growth, the mandible grows and lengthens from condylion to point B at a yearly growth rate of 1.6 mm for females and 2.2 mm for males [19]. Growth at a significantly accelerated rate or for a prolonged postpubertal time interval usually indicates active CH[19].

The diagnosis of CH may be achieved by a combination of clinical and radiologic findings. Various methods have been used, including radiographic studies, bone scintigraphy, and histopathologic assessment. Panoramic and postero-anterior (PA) radiographs are useful for surveying the shapes of the mandibular condyles on both sides because the midlines of the face and dentition can be recorded and evaluated[15]. The lateral radiograph provides useful information, such as ramal height and mandibular condyle length. CT can also provide a three-dimensional rendition of both the soft tissue of the face and the underlying bone. TMJ radiographs may show abnormalities in the size and morphology of the condylar head and/or neck regions.

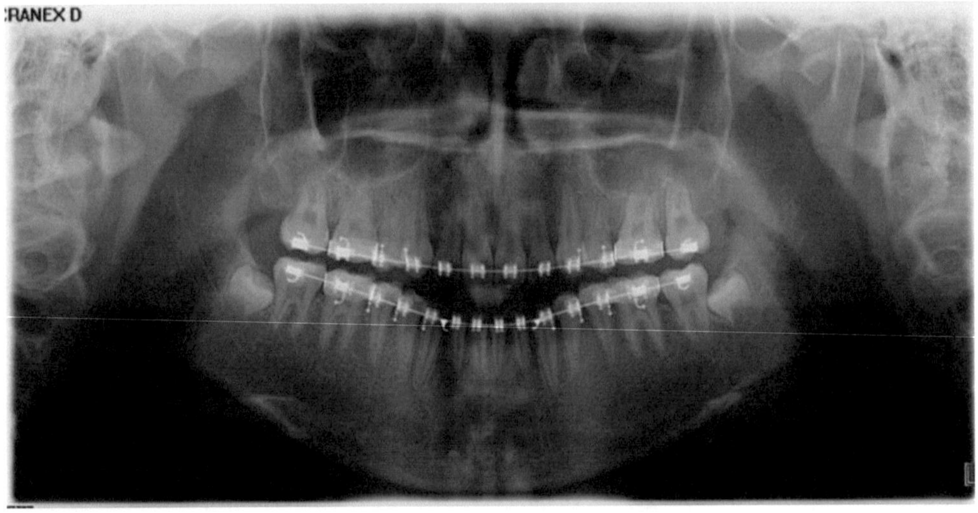

Fig. 3. Panoramic radiograph showing elongation of left condyle

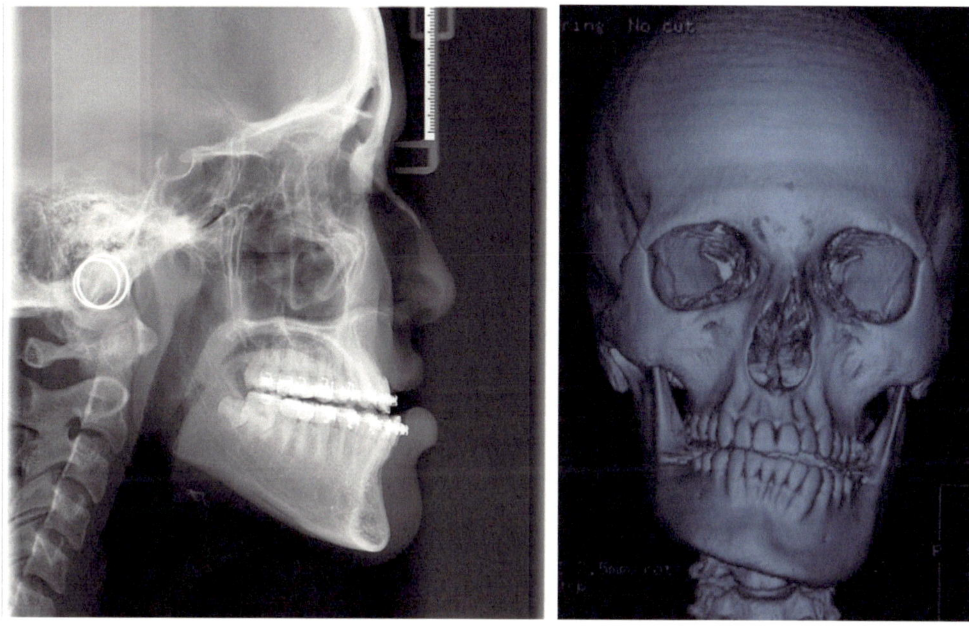

Fig. 4. Cephalogram radiograph and ct with three dimensional reconstruction

In order to develop the correct surgical plan, it is essential to distinguish active from inactive forms. Active CH growth can be determined by worsening functional and esthetic changes in time and might be detected by serial assessments consisting of clinical evaluation; dental model analysis and radiographic evaluation. Bone single photon emission computed tomography (SPECT) scan is an essential diagnostic tool for visualizing hyperactivity in the condyle[16], especially in unilateral cases. Various studies have shown the clinical significance of this technique in such patients because this method identifies those with persistent unilateral condylar activity[16]. The radioactive isotope is technetium 99 methylene bisphosphonate. Increased radionuclide uptake by the hyperplastic condyle can be an indication of continued abnormal growth[16]. It has been reported that when there is a difference in activity of 10 % or more between the two condyles, it can be indicative of CH[16]. SPECT may be most effective in unilateral cases, especially if applied after the normal growing years, when condylar growth should have ceased. It might be inconclusive in younger patients, bilateral cases and those with slow growing CH. It is important to emphasize that SPECT results should be interpreted associated with clinical, radiographic, and cephalometric evaluation[16]. It should be borne in mind that this method of bone scanning, though highly sensitive, is nonspecific and does not necessarily correlate with active growth because it can also be the result of inflammatory conditions, infection, healing after traumatic injuries, and neoplastic lesions[16]. Bone SPECT scintigraphy should not be used as the only determinant for surgical treatment[16].

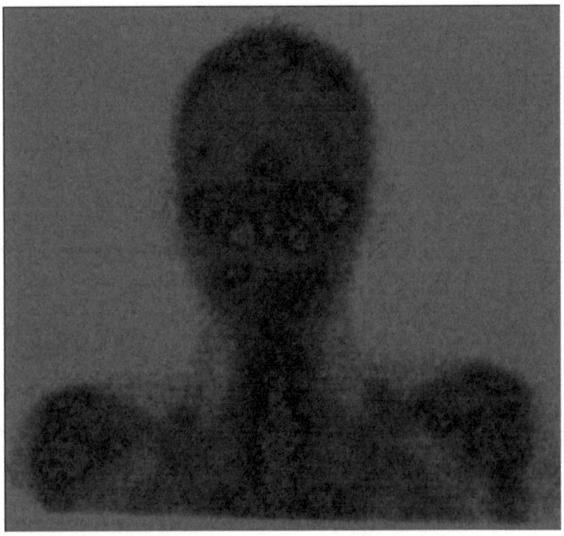

Fig. 5. Bone spect scintigraphy showing increased radionuclide uptake on left condyle

2.2 Classification and characteristics

Since 1836, when was first described by Adams[12], many cases of CH have been reported in the literature, but the key to understanding this clinical condition is attributed to Obwegeser and Makek, 1986[8]. They classified the asymmetry associated with CH into 3 categories: hemimandibular hyperplasia, causing asymmetry in the vertical plane; hemimandibular elongation, resulting in asymmetry in the transverse plane; and a combination of the 2 entities[8]. The first type is caused by unilateral growth in the vertical plane and is characterized by increased height of the maxillary alveolar bone and downward deviation of the occlusal plane in the ipsilateral side with almost no deviation of the chin[8]. If the maxillary plane fails to follow the mandibular plane, then an open bite may develop on the same side[8]. Most commonly, the mandibular midline is straight, but it may shift ipsilaterally[8]. Radiologically, Obewegeser and Makek reported that the condyle appears enlarged and that its head is usually irregular and deformed and its neck thickened and elongated, with coarse trabeculae filling the condyle[8]. Hemimandibular elongation, the second type of CH, is associated with chin deviation toward the contralateral side with no vertical asymmetry[8]. Intraorally, the mandibular midline deviates to the un-affected side, while the contralateral mandibular molars deviate lingually in attempt to remain in occlusion; however, cross-bite may develop in the contralateral side[8]. The occlusal plane is maintained with no deviation[8]. The condyle is of normal shape and size, but its neck can be either slender or normal, with an elongated ascending ramus[8]. The third type of CH is a combination of the first 2 types[8].

Wolford et. al, in 2002 and 2009, proposed a simple classification to identify the various types of CH based on the frequency of occurrence, the types of jaw deformity created, and the surgical procedures necessary to get the best treatment outcomes[14, 19]. This new classification seems to fit better the clinical findings in CH and can be correlated with planning treatment and prognosis.

The CH can be classified in two types:

- CH type 1 is the most frequently occurring form and involves an accelerated growth rate of the mandibular condyle with relatively normal architecture but elongation of the condylar head, neck, and mandibular body. It has a predominant horizontal growth vector, causing a Class III occlusal and skeletal relationship, although occasionally a vertical growth vector may occur. Type 1A is the bilateral form of CH with symmetric growth or asymmetric growth. Type 1B involves only one condyle, creating a progressively worsening facial asymmetry as the condyle growths. The accelerated mandibular growth usually occurs during puberty, and the mandibular growth can continue into the mid 20s but is self-limiting. The prevalence ratio between types 1 and 2 is approximately 15:1.
- CH type 2 occurs unilaterally and involves enlargement of the condylar head. Usually the condylar neck increases in thickness and the vertical height of the mandibular ramus and body increases on the ipsilateral side, often accompanied by a compensatory downward growth of the ipsilateral maxilla. CH type 2 can occur at any age and is not self-limiting. It can be caused by an osteochondroma, osteoma, or other rare forms of condylar enlargement.

Clinical and radiographic characteristics in CH type 1[19]
1. Increased length of the condylar head and neck, with normal architecture.
2. Accelerated rate of mandibular growth, beyond normal growth years.
3. Worsening Class III skeletal and occlusal relationship
4. Worsening aesthetics.
5. Obtuse gonial angles
6. Decreased angulation of lower incisors and increased angulation of upper incisors (dental compensations)
7. Decreased vertical height of the posterior mandibular body
8. High mandibular plane angle

Aditional clinical and radiographic characteristics in CH type 1B[19]
1. TMJ articular disc displacement on the contralateral side as a result of increased loading of that joint caused by the condylar hyperplasia on the opposite side
2. Worsening facial and occlusal asymmetry, with the mandible progres-sively shifting toward the contralateral side
3. Unilateral posterior cross-bite on the contralateral side
4. Transverse bowing of the mandibular body on the ipsilateral side
5. Transverse flattening of the mandibular body on the contralateral side

Clinical and radiographic characteristics in CH type 2[14]
1. Unilateral elongation of the face, causing facial asymmetry and worsening esthetics
2. Increased length, size, and diameter of the condylar head and neck
3. Increased vertical height of the entire mandible on the involved side (except for the coronoid process)
4. Open bite on the involved side
5. Compensatory vertical overdevelopment of the maxilla on the involved side
6. Dental compensations.

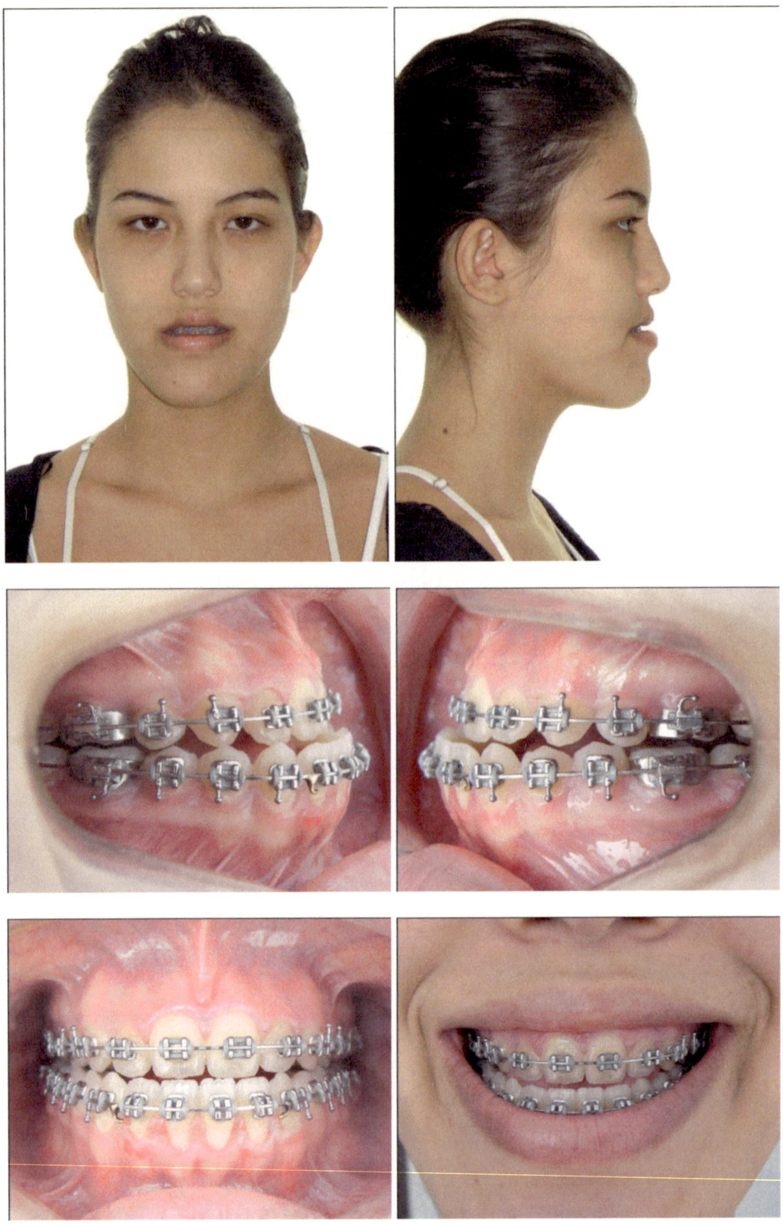

Fig. 6. CH type 1 on left condyle with facial assymetry, presenting mandibular midline deviation toward right side and right cross bite.

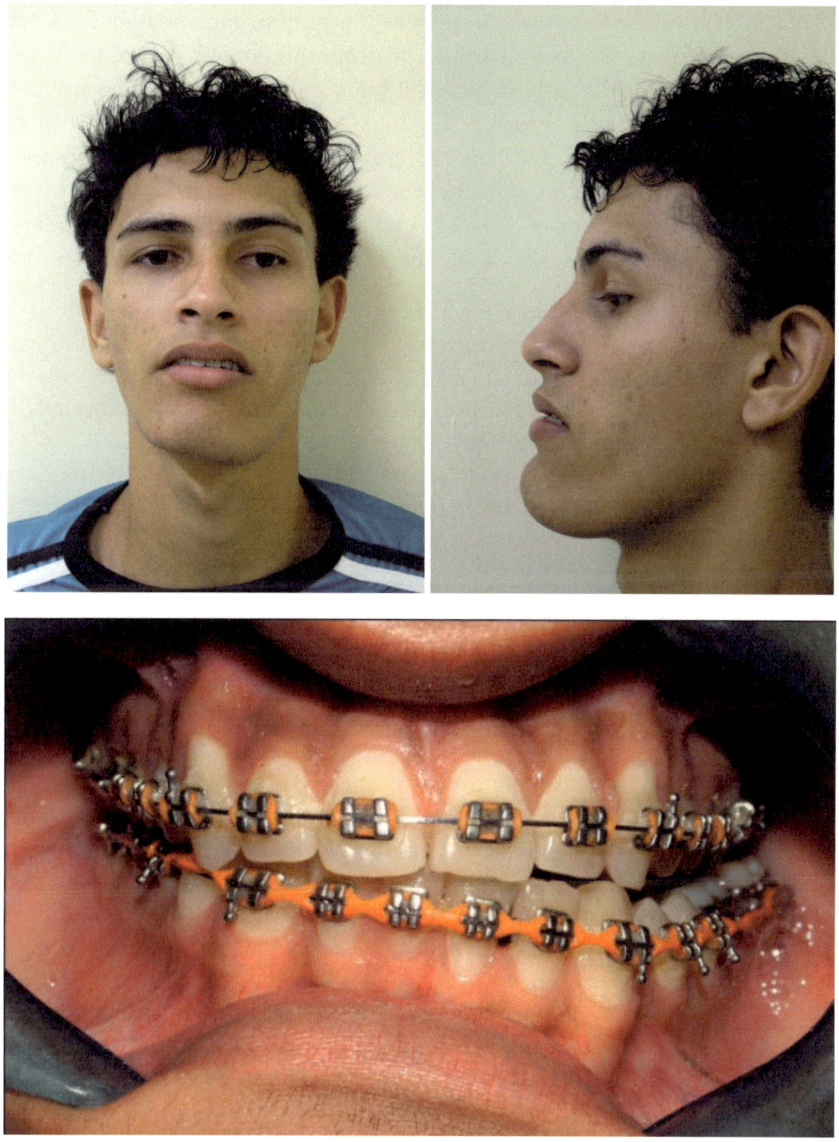

* Case provided by Dr. Elvidio de Paula e Silva

Fig. 7. CH type 2 on left condyle, presenting left elongation of mandible, left open bite and maxillary canting on left side.

2.3 Treatment planning

The treatment of CH is directly related to its activity. Patients with arrested CH (the abnormal condylar growth has stopped and become stable) can usually be treated with routine orthodontics and orthognathic surgery[14]. Treatment of active CH is primarily surgical, with or without orthodontics, and depends on the degree of severity and the status of condylar growth[16]. Different surgical options have been proposed for treating this entity, ranging from high condylectomy to orthognathic surgery or a combination of both[16]. The high condylectomy arrests the excessive and disproportionate growth of the mandible by surgically removing one of the important mandibular growth sites and the site responsible for the CH pathological growth process[19]. The high condylectomy stops forward growth of the mandible, with only normal appositional growth remaining at pogonion and vertical alveolar growth if the surgery is performed before normal facial growth is completed[20]. There is also controversy with respect to the time of surgery, with some authors preferring to perform surgery as soon as possible and others waiting for cessation of excessive activity to perform any intervention[16].

The aim in immature patients is prevention of the progression of deformities and the spontaneous normalization of facial asymmetry and occlusion. The one surgical procedure that is able to stop disease progression and allow spontaneous resolution of dento-alveolar problems is condylectomy, if performed early (10 to 12 years old). This procedure leads to the removal of the hyperactive growth center, with physiological mandibular and dento-alveolar reshaping, and consequent normalization of the face and occlusion.

In adults, most dental compensations, functional problems and facial deformities are already in development. There are some options of treatment that have been reported. Previously, some authors advocated that corrective surgery could be deferred until growth was complete; this often means waiting until the middle or late 20s[22]. In these cases, the patient might suffer from functional problems (mastication and speech), worsening esthetic disfigurement, pain, and psychosocial stigmata associated with a severe facial deformity. Additionally, the magnitude of the deformity, if allowed to fully manifest by this delay in treatment, may preclude an ideal result later. This hyperplastic condylar growth may result in severe deformation of the mandible. Compensatory changes will occur in the maxilla, dentoalveolar structures, and associated soft tissue structures, significantly compromising the clinical treatment outcome. This treatment has been advocated by many surgeons in previous reports. However, with the full comprehensive of progression of CH and its consequences, it doesn´t seems to be a good choice. Other authors have reported that orthognathic surgery could be performed during active CH growth, with consideration for overcorrection of the mandible. The accelerated mandibular condylar growth will continue after surgery, and repeat surgery will be needed if the estimated overcorrection is greater or lesser than necessary.

Based on surgical results of previous reports[14,19] and many reports of bad results with other techniques[14], is believed that the two best treatment options for achieving favorable functional and esthetics results, with long-term stability are as follows:

1. The high condilectomy with disc repositioning is performed as soon as possible to arrest condyle and mandibular growth. Then, the orthodontic treatment aims to align and level the teeth over the basal bone and to remove dental compensations, regardless of the magnitude of skeletal and dental malalignment. In a second staged surgery, the conventional orthognathic surgery is performed. Usually, due to severe skeletal and dental deformity, bimaxillary surgery is necessary to achieve both functional and esthetic results. This treatment might be the choice when the orthodontic treatment will delay the condilectomy, with worsening of face and dental deformity.

2. The high condylectomy with disc repositioning is performed with simultaneous orthognathic surgery. This technique is helpful when patients have passed through orthodontic treatment previously and would be benefit with on staged surgery. The benefits of concomitant surgery provided to patients with coexisting TMJ pathology and dentofacial deformities include the following: 1) that it requires one operation and general anesthetic; 2) that it balances occlusion, TMJs, jaws, and neuromuscular structures, at the same time; 3) that it decreases overall treatment time; 4) that it eliminates unfavorable TMJ sequelae that can occur when performing orthognathic surgery only; and 5) that it avoids iatrogenic malocclusion that can occur when performing open TMJ surgery only[21].

In CH type 2, the treatment is similar as described above. However, in cases of condylar enlargement by ostoeocondromas or other benign tumors, it might be necessary a more aggressive approach, with total resection of the tumor and reconstruction with autogenus grafts or total joint prosthesis. Traditional treatment of almost all reported cases of osteochondroma has included radical resection of the tumor, including the complete condylar process[23,24,25]. Free autogenous bone grafts, costochondral grafts, prosthetic devices, or local pedicled osseous grafts have been used to reconstruct the TMJ region[26]. Wolford et. al, 2002, proposed a conservative condylectomy below the head but high in the neck of the condyle, to entirely remove the lesion[27]. The remaining condylar stump is recontourned to function as a "new" condylar head. The articular disc is then repositioned onto the "new" condyle and stabilized[27]. Additional orthognathic procedures, if indicated, can be performed concomitantly for the correction of associated facial deformities[27].

Classification	Treatment
Arrested CH	Orthodontics and orthognathic surgery
Active CH in infants	High condylectomy and observation
Active CH in adults	High condylectomy and orthognathic surgery in one or two stages
CH type 2	Condylectomy and orthognatic surgery OR Condylar resection and total joint reconstruction*.

* in cases of large osteocondromas or other benign tumors.

Table 1. Surgical techinque

The surgical approach to TMJ structures is pre-auricular approach. The incision is marked on intersection of pre-auricular facial skin and ear helix. After preoperative drawing and landmark placement, a cutaneous incision is performed and deepened until reaching the deep temporal fascia. The superficial layer of the deep fascia is cut, reaching the fat tissue between the two layers of the temporal fascia[28]. The dissection is proceeded deeper to the superficial layer of the fascia and reached the TMJ capsule caudal to the zygomatic arch. This is opened with a "T" incision, which identify the condylar head and disc. The condylar head is gently split from the articular disc, and condylar protectors are set medially to the head. A horizontal osteotomy line is drawn 4 e 5 mm caudal to the edge of the condylar head. The osteotomy is completed with chisel, the resected part is removed and the surface of the condylar head reshaped. Then, the articular disc is repositioned on condylar surface and attached with mini anchors or mini screws.

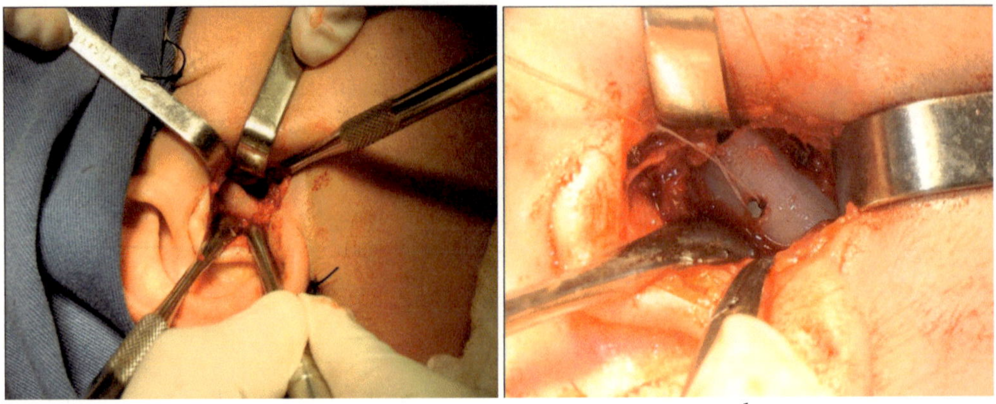

a b

Fig. 8. Surgical exposure of right condyle (a) and high condylectomy with disc repositioning with mini-anchors (b).

If bimaxillary orthognathic surgery is planned to be performed concomitant with TMJ surgery, 2 choices of sequencing are possible. The first sequence will follow maxilla repositioning first, TMJ surgery, and then the mandibular osteotomy. The second sequence would be to first perform the TMJ surgery, then the mandibular osteotomy, and then to reposition the maxilla. Both techniques can provide the same results[30]. However, the first sequence would make it much more difficult to maintain sterility during the TMJ surgery[30]. One would have to try and maintain separate surgical fields (TMJ and oral cavity) and have a second set of sterile instruments available for the TMJ surgery[30]. When performing TMJ surgery first, the same set of instruments used for the TMJ can be used for the mandibular and, subsequently, maxillary surgery[30].

2.4 3-Dimensional (3D) surgical planning and use of navigation

To facilitate the estimation of condylectomy and other mandibular contouring surgeries, 3-dimensional (3D) surgical planning by use of computed tomography (CT) data is now available and can be extremely helpful[31]. Surgical planning can be performed either with a stereolithographic or a virtual model generated by commercial softwares[31]. Surgical navigation is preferred as data export, because the surgical splint is considered bulky for precise placement during condylectomy and contouring surgeries[31]. Although various options are available for surgical planning and simulation, a precise data transfer to the real surgical environment still appears to be challenging to surgeons[31]. Currently, there are 2 approaches available for such a transfer: 1) surgical locating splint and; 2) real-time surgical navigation.

The surgical splint can be generated either from 1) a stereolithographic model planning with the help from laboratory technicians or 2) a virtual model planning by use of computer-aided design/computer-aided manufacturing technology[31]. The stereolitho-graphic model planning is a relatively straightforward approach[31]. However, the seating of a surgical splint is highly dependent on sound anatomic structure with well-defined surface geometry for its fitting[31]. In situations such as condylectomy and mandibuloplasty, splint placement may be complicated because of limited surgery access[30]. Although surgical navigation allows location of the drilling path under standard surgical exposure, the use in the mandible is handicapped because of its mobile nature[30]. By combining the merits of surgical navigation and stereolithographic model planning, Xia et. al (2010) have formulated a new treatment strategy, which involves correction of occlusal disharmony and skeletal deformity in one operation with a shorter time[31]. In the appropriate delegation of responsibility, surgeons need to prepare the model surgery planning and the transfer of the model surgery data to the surgical navigation system.

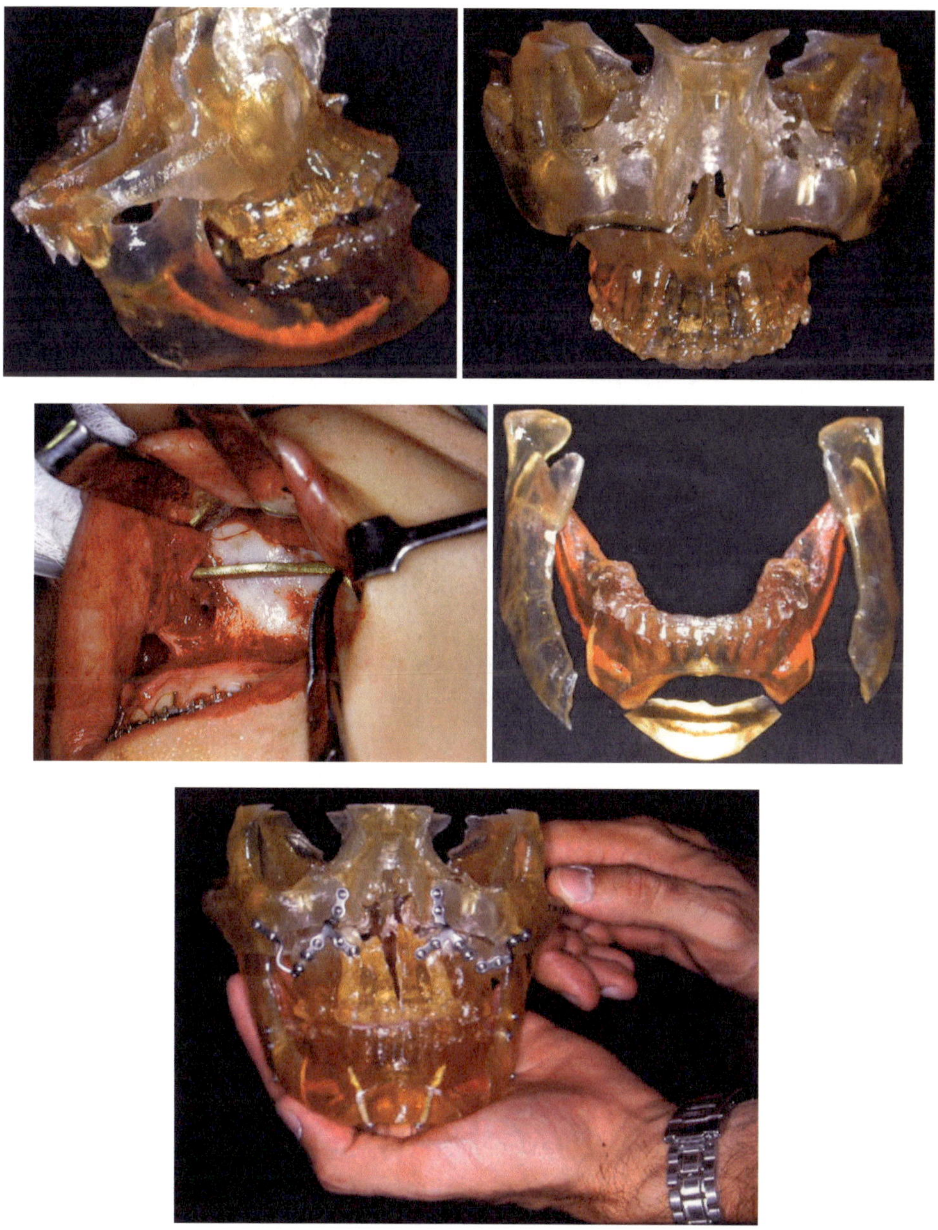

Fig. 9. Treatment planning using surgical simulation on a stereolithographic provided by Dr. Cesar Oleskovicz.

3. Case presentation

3.1 Case 1

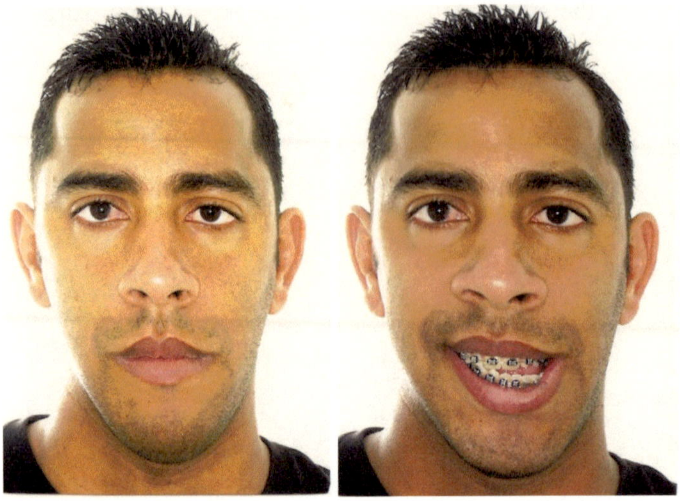

Fig. 10. Initial front and profile view

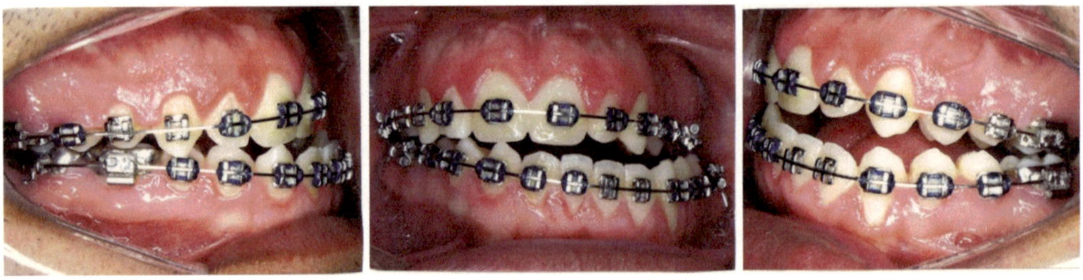

Fig. 11. Presurgical occlusion

LIST OF PROBLEMS	TREATMENT PLAN
Facial asymmetry	Surgically assisted rapid palatal expansion (SARME) - First surgery
Class III malocclusion	Presurgical orthodontic treatment
CH type 1 on right side with horizontal and vertical growth vector	High condylectomy with orthognathic surgery
Transverse maxillary deficiency and canting on left side	Le Fort I osteotomy with superior repositioning and maxillary advancement and leveling.
Open bite	Mandibular advancement with superior and forward repositioning genioplasty.
Cross bite on left side	
Vertical excess of lower face	

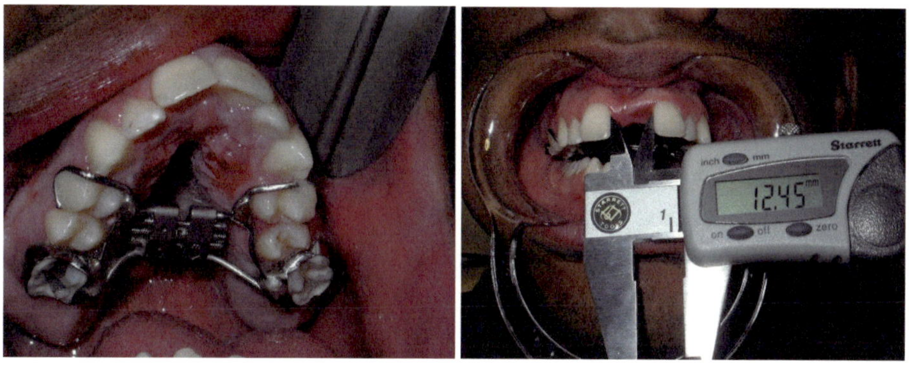

Fig. 12. First surgery - surgically assisted rapid palatal expansion (sarme)

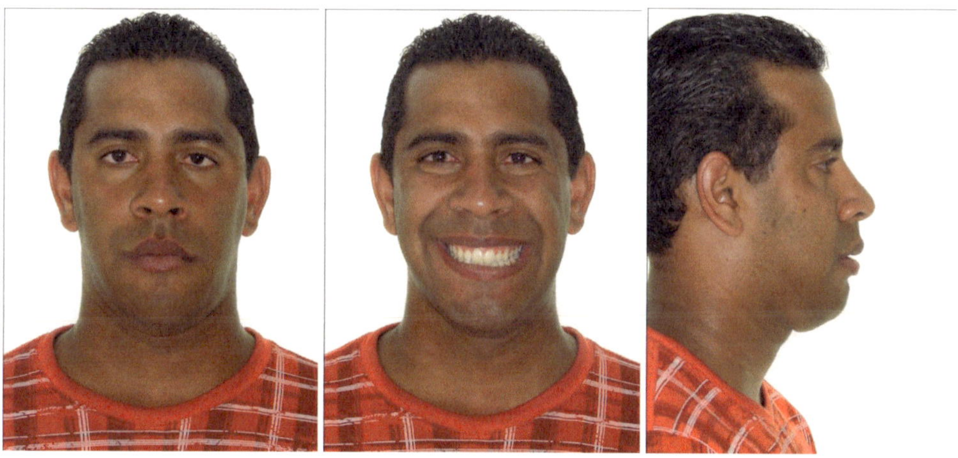

Fig. 13. Final frontal and profile view

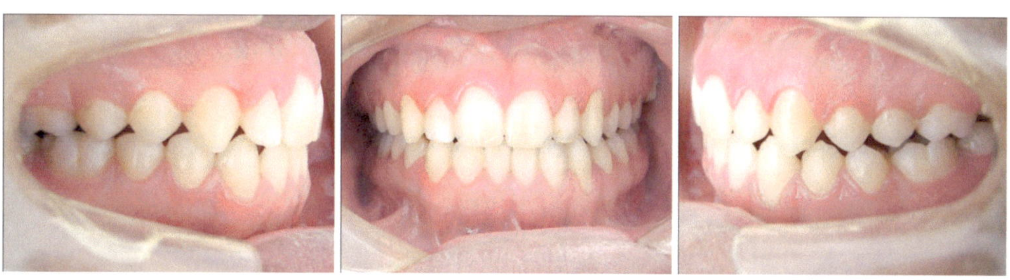

Fig. 14. Final occlusion

3.2 Case 2

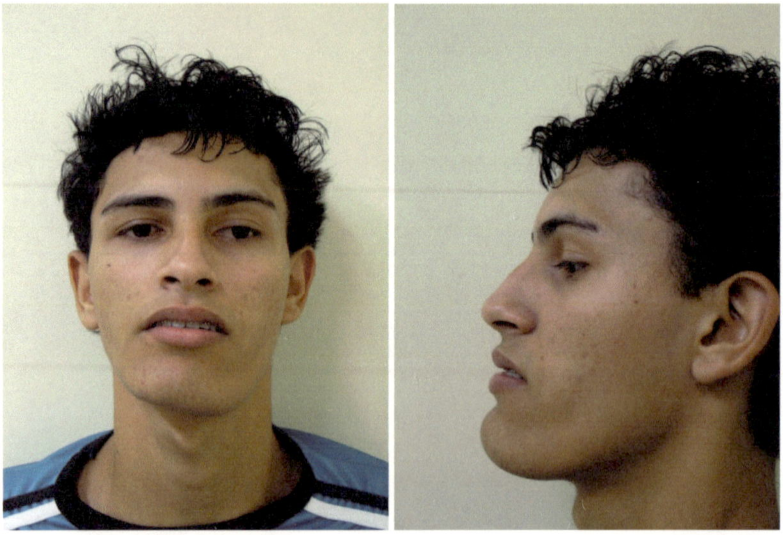

Fig. 15. Inicial frontal and profile view

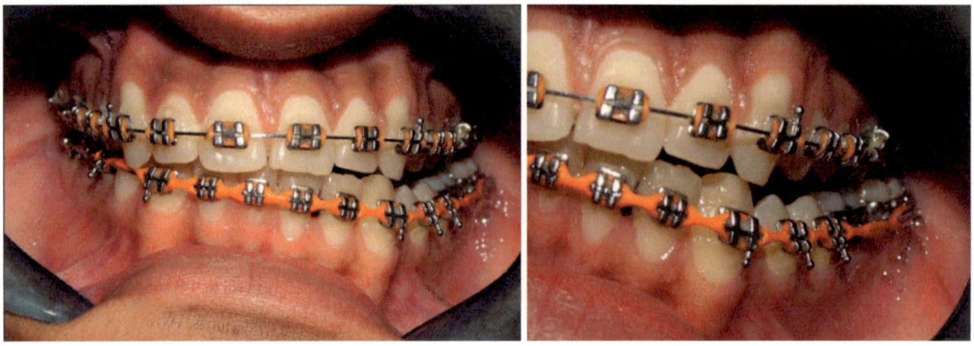

Fig. 16. Pretreatment occlusion

LIST OF PROBLEMS	TREATMENT PLAN
Facial asymmetry	High condylectomy and mandibular osteoplasty on left body and chin
Class III malocclusion	Presurgical othodontic treatment
CH type 2 on left side with mandibular midline deviation towards left side	Le Fort I osteotomy with maxillary advancement and leveling
Maxillary canting on left side	Mandibular setback with superior repositioning and setback genioplasty
Cross bite on left side	
Vertical excess of chin	

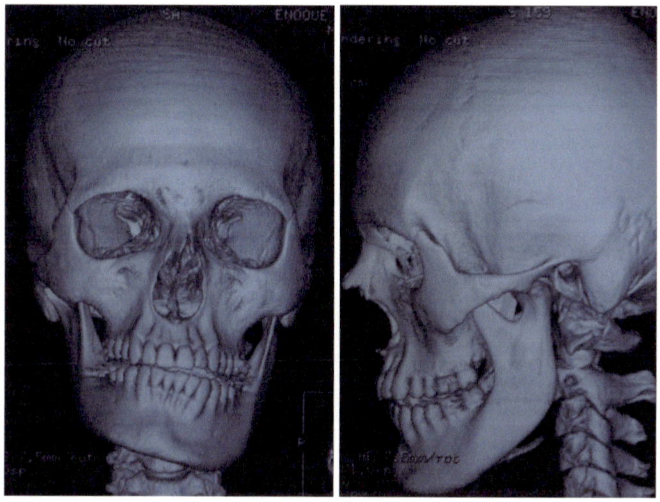

Fig. 17. CT images showing left condyle enlargment

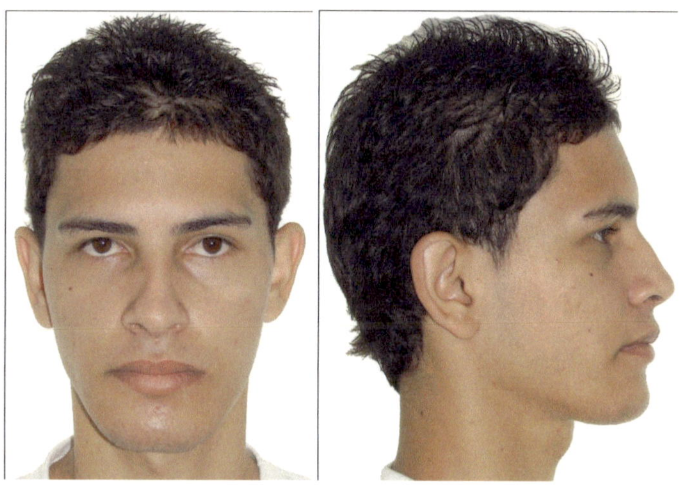

Fig. 18. Final front and profile view

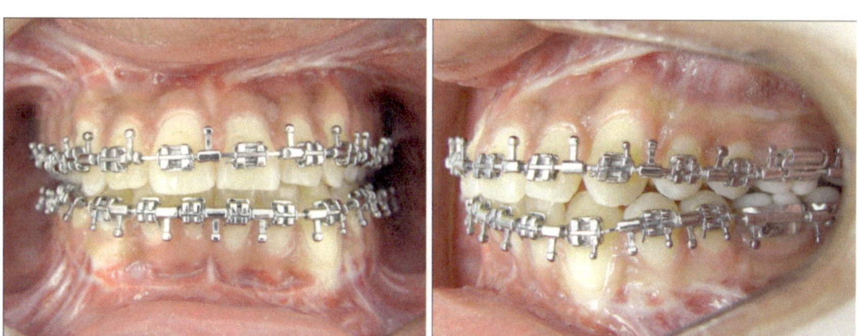

* Case provided by Dr. Elvidio de Paula e Silva

Fig. 19. Final occlusion

3.3 Case 3

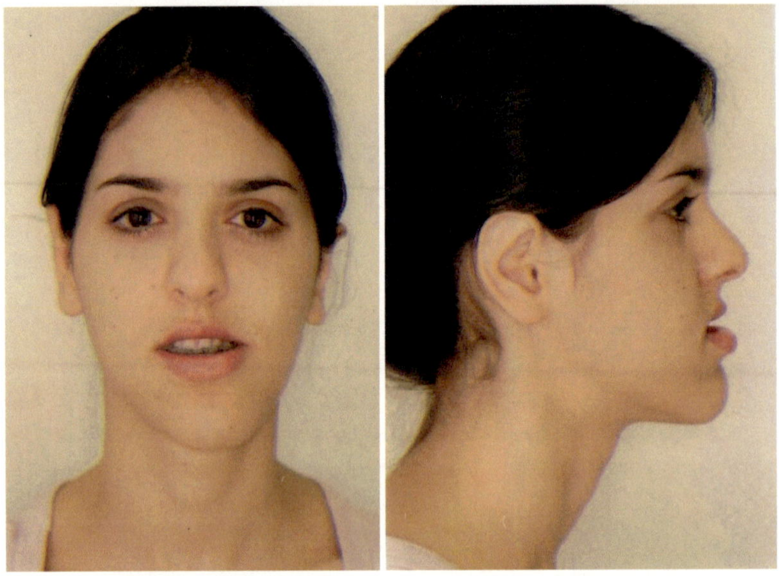

Fig. 20. Initial front and profile view

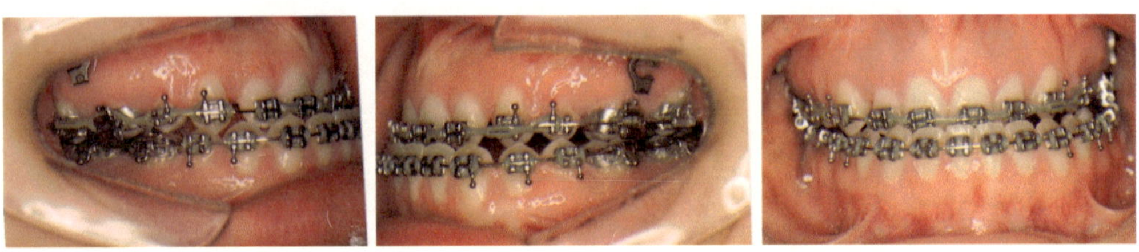

Fig. 21. Initial occlusion

LIST OF PROBLEMS	TREATMENT PLAN
Facial asymmetry	Presurgical orthodontic treatment
Class III malocclusion	High condilectomy with orthognathic surgery
CH type 1 on right side with midline deviation towards left side	Le Fort I osteotomy with superior repositioning and maxillary advancement and leveling.
Anterior cross bite	Mandibular setback with superior and forward repositioning genioplasty.
Cross bite on left side	
Vertical excess of chin	

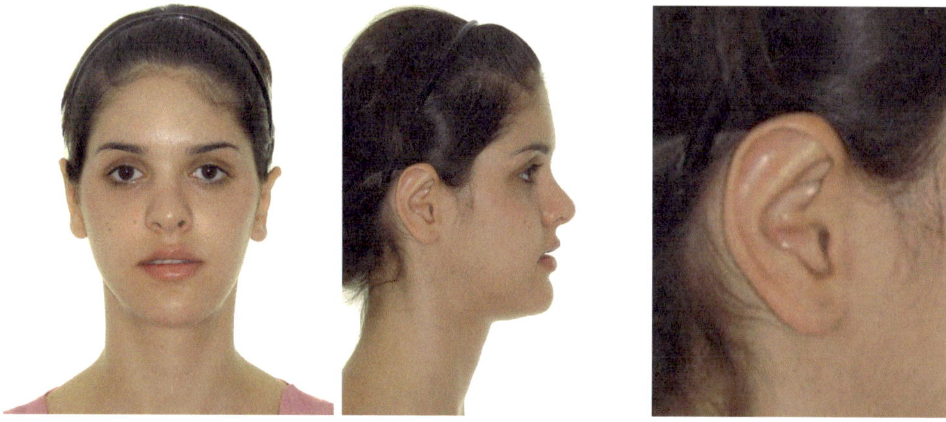

Fig. 22. Final front and profile view and preauricular region showing small residual scar

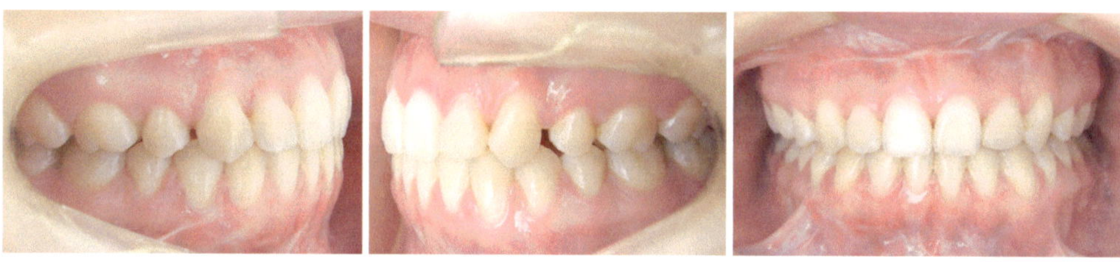

Fig. 23. Final occlusion

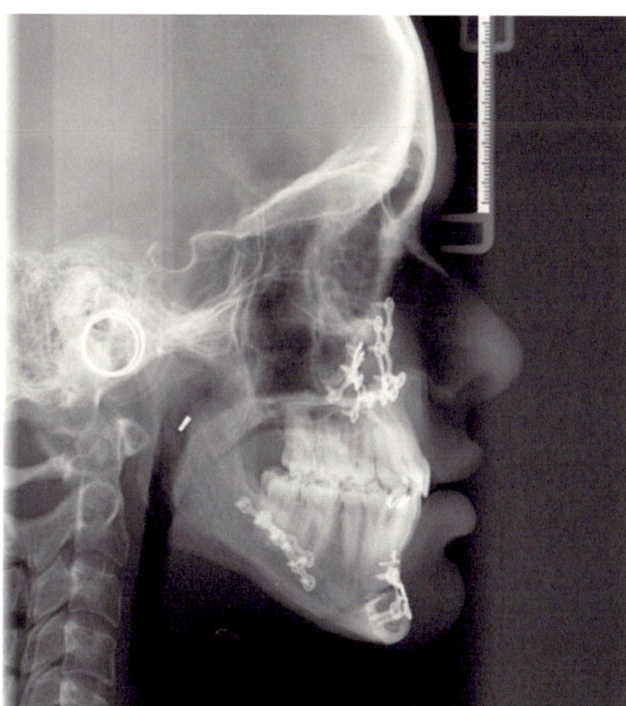

Fig. 24. Final cephalogram radiographs

3.4 Case 4

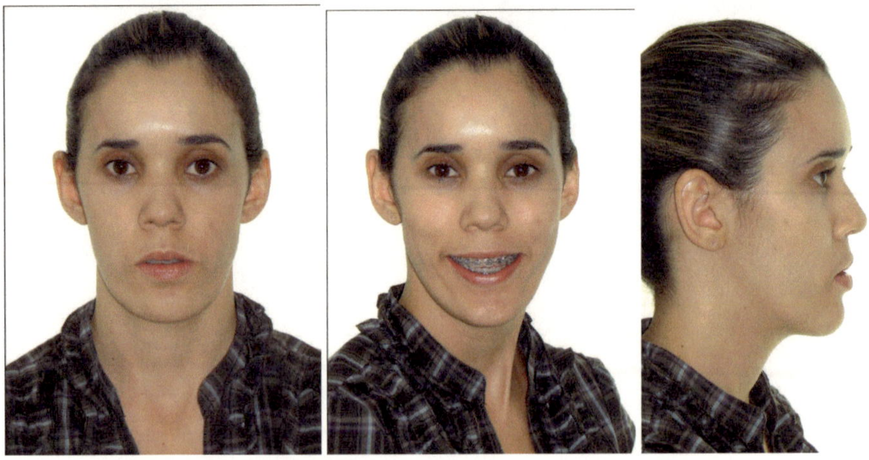

Fig. 25. Initial front and profile view (above) and initial occlusal (bellow)

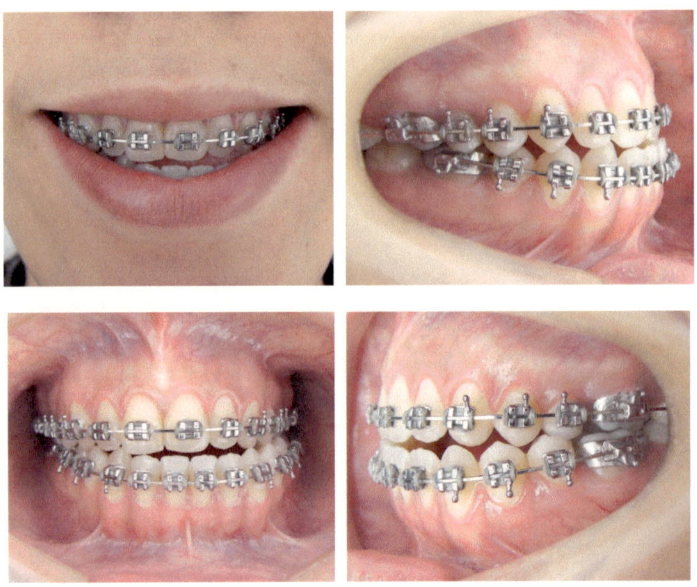

LIST OF PROBLEMS	TREATMENT PLAN
Facial asymmetry	Presurgical orthodontic treatment
Class III malocclusion	High condilectomy with orthognathic surgery
CH type 1 on right side with mandibular midline deviation towards left side	Le Fort I osteotomy with superior repositioning and maxillary advancement and leveling.
Maxillary midline deviation towards right side	Mandibular setback with superior and forward repositioning genioplasty.
Cross bite on left side	Augmentation of left mandibular angle with a high-density polyethylene implant (MEDPOR®)
Vertical excess of chin	
Flattening of left mandibular angle	

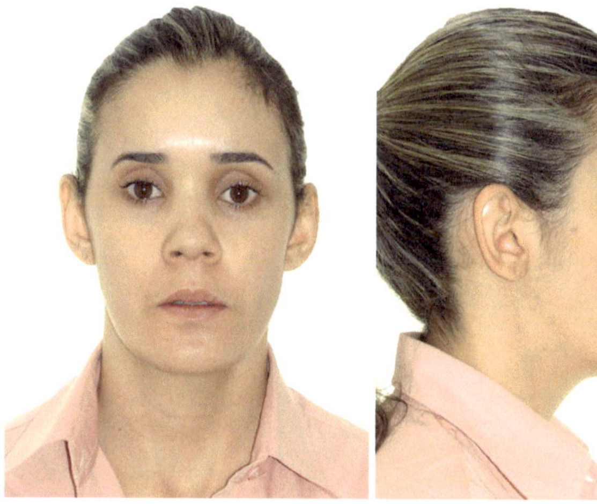

Fig. 26. Final frontal and profile view one year after surgery

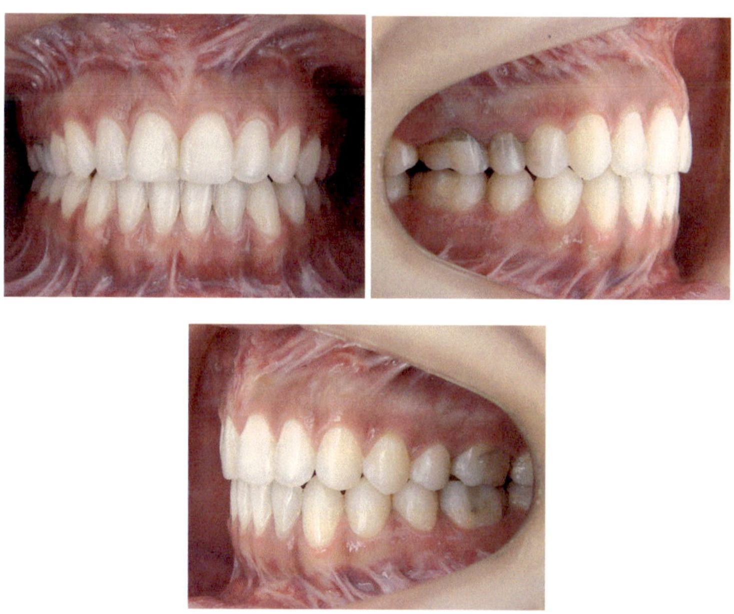

Fig. 27. Final occlusion

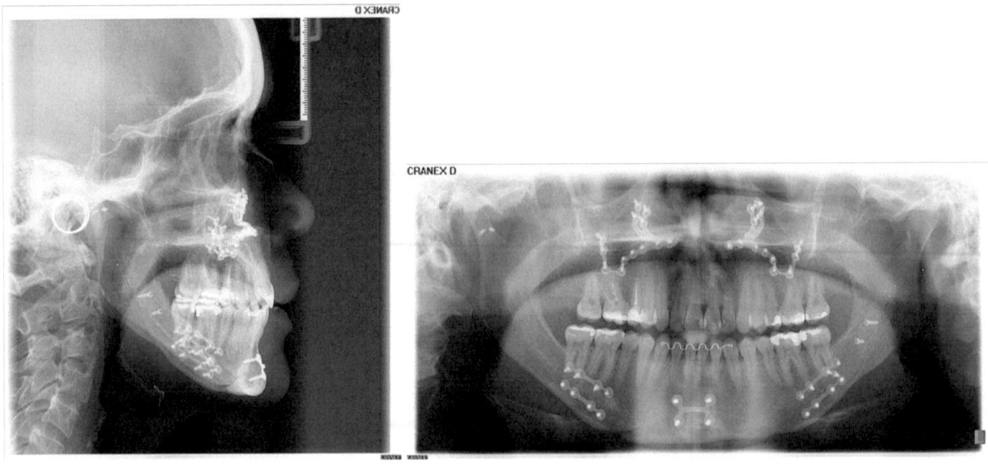

Fig. 28. Final cephalogram and panoramic radiographs showing mini-anchors on right condyle

4. Conclusions

Treatment of facial asymmetry can be challenging for both orthodontists and oral and maxillofacial surgeons. They can be assessed by photographs, posteroanterior cephalograms and 3D computed tomography (CT) scans, but clinical examinations is mandatory in order to obtain optimal functional and aesthetics results.

Mandibular condylar hiperplasia with active growth represents an important role in facial asymmetry and its treatment can be achieved by correct diagnosis, orthodontic treatment associated with correct surgical techniques.

5. References

[1] Ko,E.W.C; Huang,C.S.; Chen, Y.R.J. Characteristics and Corrective Outcome of Face Asymmetry by Orthognathic Surgery. J Oral Maxillofac Surg 67:2201-2209, 2009.

[2] Lee, M.; Chung, D.H; Lee, J.; Cha, K. Assessing soft-tissue characteristics of facial asymmetry with photographs. Am J Orthod Dentofacial Orthop; 138:23-31, 2010.

[3] Bishara SE, Burkey PS, Kharouf JG. Dental and facial asymmetries: a review. Angle Orthod 1994;64:89-98.

[4] Hwang, H-S; Youn, S.; Lee, K-H; Lim, H-J. Classification of facial asymmetry by cluster analysis. Am J Orthod Dentofacial Orthop; 132:279.e1-279.e6; 2007.

[5] Hinds EC, Reid LC, Burch RJ. Classification and management of mandibular asymmetry. Am J Surg 1960;100:825-34.

[6] Rowe NL. Aetiology, clinical features, and treatment of mandib-ular deformity. Br Dent J 1960;108:64-96.

[7] Bruce RA, Hayward JR. Condylar hyperplasia and mandibular asymmetry: a review. J Oral Surg 1968;26:281-90.

[8] Obwegeser HL, Makek MS. Hemimandibular hyperplasia—hemimandibular elongation. J Maxillofac Surg 1986;14:183-208;

[9] Padwa, B.L; Kaiser, M.O; Kaban, L.B. Occlusal Cant in the Frontal Plane as a Reflection of Facial Asymmetry. J Oral Maxiliofac Surg, 55:811-816, 1997.

[10] New Clinical Protocol to Evaluate Craniomaxillofacial Deformity and Plan Surgical Correction. Xia, J.J; Gateno, J.; Teichgraeber, J.F. J Oral Maxillofac Surg, 67:2093-2106, 2009.

[11] Iannetti, G.; Cascone, P.; Belli, E.; Cordaro, L. Condylar hiperplasia: Cephalometric study, treatment plannin, and surgical correction (our experience). Oral Surg Olar Med Oral Pathol; 68:673-81, 1989.

[12] Adams R. The disease in the temporomandibular articulation or joint of the lower jaw. In A Treatise on Rheumatic Gout or Chronic Rheumatic Arthritis of All the Joints, 2nd ed. London: Churchill, 1873:271.

[13] Nitzan, D.W.; Katsnelson, A.; Bermanis, I.; Brin, I; Casap, N. The Clinical Characteristics of Condylar Hyperplasia: Experience With 61 Patients. J Oral Maxillofac Surg 66:312-318, 2008

[14] Wolford LM, Mehra P, Reiche-Fischel O, Morales-Ryan CA, Garcia-Mo-rales P. Efficacy of high condylectomy for management of condylar hyper-plasia. Am J Orthod Dentofacial Orthop 2002;121(2):136–150

[15] Kaneyama, K.; Segami, N.; Hatta, N. Congenital deformities and developmental abnormalities of the mandibular condyle in the temporomandibular joint Congenital Anomalies 2008; 48, 118–125.

[16] Villanueva-Alcojol, L.; Monje, F.; González-García, R. Hyperplasia of the Mandibular Condyle: Clinical, Histopathologic, and Treatment Considerations in a Series of 36 Patients J Oral Maxillofac Surg 69:447-455, 2011

[17] Norman JE, Painter DM: Hyperplasia of the mandibular condyle: A historical review of important early cases with a presentation and analysis of twelve patients. J Maxillofac Surg 8:161, 1980.

[18] Saridin, C.P; Raijmakers, P.G.H.M.; Slootweg, P.J; Tuinzing, D.B.; Becking, A.G.; van der Waa, I. Unilateral Condylar Hyperactivity: A Histopathologic Analysis of 47 Patients J Oral Maxillofac Surg 68:47-53, 2010.

[19] Surgical management of mandibular condylar hyperplasia type 1. Wolford LM, Morales-Ryan CA, García-Morales P, Perez D. Proc (Bayl Univ Med Cent). 2009 Oct;22(4):321-9.

[20] Brusati, R..; Pedrazzo, M.; Colletti, G. Functional results after condylectomy in active laterognathia. Journal of Cranio-Maxillo-Facial Surgery (2010) 38 , 179e184

[21] Wolford, L.M. Concomitant Temporomandibular Joint and Orthognathic Surgery. J Oral Maxillofac Surg 61:1198-1204, 2003.

[22] Marchetti C, Cocchi R, Gentile L, Bianchi A: Hemimandibular hyperplasia: treatment strategies. J Craniofac Surg 11: 46e 53, 2000

[23] Karras SC, Wolford LM, Cottrell DA: Concurrent osteochon-droma of the mandibular condyle and ipsilateral cranial base resulting in TMJ ankylosis: Report of a case and review of the literature. J Oral Maxillofac Surg 54:640, 1996

[24] Schajowicz F, Ackerman LV, Sissons HA: International Histo-logical Classification of Tumors. No. 6. Histological Typing of Bone Tumors. Geneva, Switzerland, World Health Organiza-tion, 1972

[25] Koga K, Toyama M, Kurita K: Osteochondroma of the mandib-ular angle: Report of a case. J Oral Maxillofac Surg 54:510, 1996

[26] Iizuka T, Schroth G, Laeng RH, et al: Osteochondroma of the mandibular condyle. J Oral Maxillofac Surg 54:495, 1996
[27] Wolford, L.M.; Mehra, P.; Franco, P. Use of Conservative Condylectomy for Treatment of Osteochondroma of the Mandibular Condyle. J Oral Maxillofac Surg 60:262-268, 2002
[28] Al-Kayat A, Bramley P: A modified pre-auricular approach to the temporomandibular joint and malar arch. Br J Oral Surg 17(2):91e103, 1979
[29] Perez, D.; Ellis III, E. Sequencing Bimaxillary Surgery: Mandible First. J Oral Maxillofac Surg. Article in press.
[30] Lo, J.; Xia, J.J; Zwahlen, R.A.; Cheung, L.K. Surgical Navigation in Correction of Hemimandibular Hyperplasia: A New Treatment Strategy. J Oral Maxillofac Surg 68:1444-1450, 2010

5

The Mandibular Nerve: The Anatomy of Nerve Injury and Entrapment

M. Piagkou[1], T. Demesticha[2], G. Piagkos[3], Chrysanthou Ioannis[4], P. Skandalakis[5] and E.O. Johnson[6]
[1,3,4,5,6]Department of Anatomy,
[2]Department of Anesthesiology, Metropolitan Hospital
Medical School, University of Athens
Greece

1. Introduction

The trigeminal nerve (TN) is a mixed cranial nerve that consists primarily of sensory neurons. It exists the brain on the lateral surface of the pons, entering the trigeminal ganglion (TGG) after a few millimeters, followed by an extensive series of divisions. Of the three major branches that emerge from the TGG, the mandibular nerve (MN) comprises the 3rd and largest of the three divisions. The MN also has an additional motor component, which may run in a separate facial compartment. Thus, unlike the other two TN divisions, which convey afferent fibers, the MN also contains motor or efferent fibers to innervate the muscles that are attached to mandible (muscles of mastication, the mylohyoid, the anterior belly of the digastric muscle, the tensor veli palatini, and tensor tympani muscle). Most of these fibers travel directly to their target tissues. Sensory axons innervate skin on the lateral side of the head, tongue, and mucosal wall of the oral cavity. Some sensory axons enter the mandible to innervate the teeth and emerge from the mental foramen to innervate the skin of the lower jaw.

An entrapment neuropathy is a nerve lesion caused by pressure or mechanical irritation from some anatomic structures next to the nerve. This occurs frequently where the nerve passes through a fibro-osseous canal, or because of impingement by an anatomic structure (bone, muscle or a fibrous band), or because of the combined influences on the nerve entrapment between soft and hard tissues. Any mechanical injury of the nerve therefore could be considered a compression or entrapment neuropathy **(Kwak et al., 2003).** A usual position of TN compression is the ITF **(Nayak et al., 2008),** a deep retromaxillary space, situated below the middle cranial fossa of the skull, the pharynx and the mandibular ramus. The ITF contains several of the mastication muscles, the pterygoid venous plexus, the maxillary artery (MA) and the MN ramification **(Prades et al., 2003) (Figure 1).** The MA is in contact with the inferior alveolar nerve (IAN) and lingual nerve (LN) **(Trost et al., 2009).** Recently, it is believed that some cases of temporomandibular joint syndrome (TMJS), persistent idiopathic facial pain (PIFP) and myofascial pain syndrome (MPS) may be due to entrapment neuropathies of the MN in the ITF **(Loughner et al., 1990).** Various muscle anomalies in the ITF have been reported when considering unexplained neurological symptoms attributed to MN branches. The variations of the typical nerve course are important for adequate local anaesthesia, dental, oncological and reconstructive operations **(Akita et al., 2001).** Whenever observed these variations must be reported as they can cause serious implications in any surgical intervention in the region, and may lead to false neurological differential diagnosis. If anomalous MN branches occur in combination with the ossified ligaments, then cutaneous sensory fibres might pass through one of the foramina formed by the ossified bars **(Shaw, 1993).** The MN can be compressed as a result of both its course and its relation to the surrounding structures, particularly when passing between the medial pterygoid (MPt) and lateral pterygoid (LPt) muscles. When the pterygoid muscles contract, both the IAN and the LN may be compressed. This results in pain, particularly during chewing; and may eventually cause trigeminal neuralgia (TGN) **(Anil et al., 2003).** MN entrapment can lead to numbness of all peripheral regions innervated from it. It could also lead to pain during speech **(Peuker et al., 2001).**

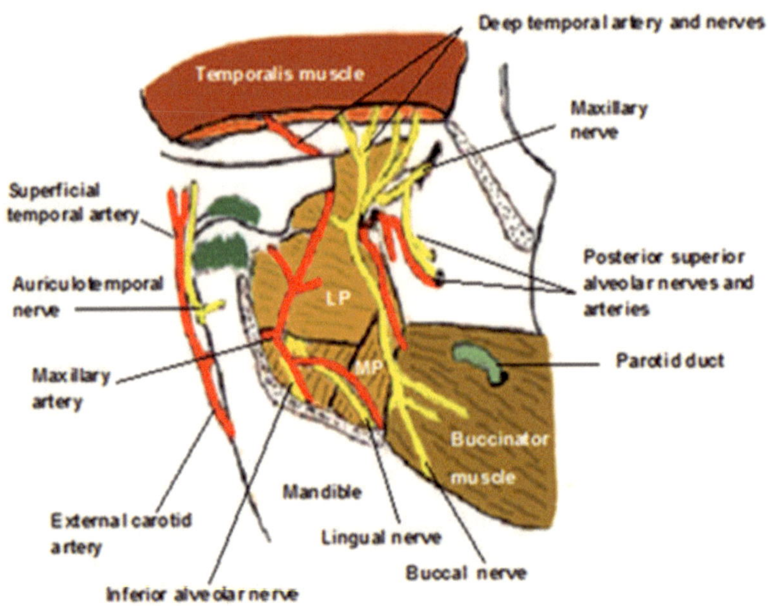

Fig. 1. The distribution of the mandibular nerve and its branches in the infratemporal fossa (ITF)

2. Typical course of mandibular nerve and its branches

The MN, the largest of the three divisions of the TN, leaves the skull through the foramen ovale (FO) and enters the ITF and medial to the LPt; it divides into a smaller anterior trunk and a larger posterior trunk. The anterior trunk passes between the roof of the ITF and the LPt and the posterior trunk descends medially to the LPt, which might entrap the nerve **(Isberg et al., 1987; Loughner et al., 1990) (Figure 2).**

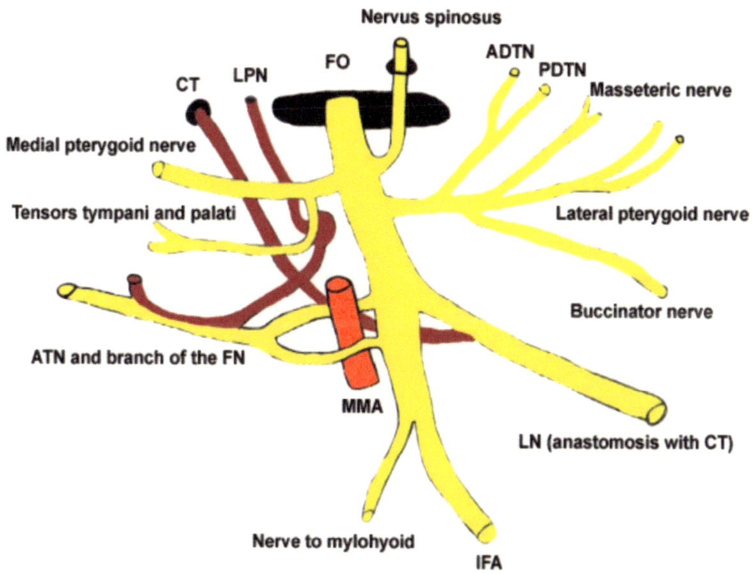

Fig. 2. The mandibular division of the TN emerging for the Foramen Ovale deep in the ITF.

3. The anterior trunk of the MN

The Buccal Nerve (BN) mainly supplies the LPt while passing through it and may give off the Anterior Deep Temporal Nerve (ADTN). It supplies the skin over the anterior part of the buccinator and the buccal mucous membrane, together with the posterior part of the buccal gingivae, adjacent to the 2nd and 3rd molar teeth. It proceeds between the two parts of the LPt, descending deep then anteriorly to the tendon of the temporalis muscle. This normal course is a potential site of entrapment. If LPt spasm occurs, the BN could be compressed, and this compression could provoke in cheek numbness. BN compression has been reported by a hyperactive temporalis muscle and may result in neuralgia-like paroxysmal pain **(Loughner al., 1990). Kim et al (2003)** found that in 8 cadavers (33.3%) the BN was entrapped within the anterior muscle fibres of the temporalis.

The Masseteric nerve passes laterally, above the LPt, on the skull base, anterior to the TMJ and posterior to the tendon of the temporalis; it crosses the posterior part of the mandibular coronoid notch with the masseteric artery, ramifies on, and enters the deep surface of masseter. It also supplies the TMJ. Compression of the masseteric nerve anterior to the TMJ was found in 1 joint with excessive condylar translation **(Johansson et al., 1990).**

The Deep temporal nerves (DTN) usually an anterior and a posterior branch pass above the LPt to enter the deep surface of the temporalis. The small Posterior Deep Temporal Nerve (PDTN) sometimes arises in common with the masseteric nerve. The Anterior Deep Temporal Nerve (ADTN), a branch of the BN, ascends over the upper head of the LPt. A middle branch often occurs. **Johannson et al. (1990)** found that the DPTN may pass close to the anterior insertion of the joint capsule on the temporal bone, exposing them to the risk of mechanical irritation in condylar hypermobility. **Loughner et al. (1990)** observed the mylohyoid nerve and ADTN passing through the LPt. A spastic condition of the LPt may be causally related to compression of an entrapped nerve that leads to numbness, pain or both in the respective nerve distribution areas. *Compression of sensory branches* of the DTN by the temporalis muscle is a cause of neuropathy, (neuralgia or paresthesia) neuralgia or paresthesia **(Madhavi et al., 2006).**

The Nerve to the LPt enters the deep surface of the muscle and may arise separately from the anterior division or with the BN.

4. The posterior trunk of the MN

The Auriculotemporal Nerve (ATN) usually has 2 roots, arising from the posterior division of MN. It encircles the middle meningeal artery (MMA) and runs posteriorly passing between the sphenomandibular ligament (SML) and the neck of the mandible. It then runs laterally behind the TMJ to emerge deep in the upper part of the parotid gland. The nerve carries somatosensory and secremotor fibres of the MN and the glossopharyngeal nerve (GPhN). The ATN communicates with the facial nerve (FN) at the posterior border of the ramus where the ATN passes posterior to the neck of the condyle. If fibres cross over from the ATN to the FN and not vice versa, this communication may represent a pathway for FN sensory impairment; i.e. pain in the muscles of facial expression may occur due to an entrapped and compressed ATN. An entrapped ATN in the LPt could be the aetiology behind a painful neuropathy in a distal ATN branch supplying sensory innervation to a deranged TMJ **(Akita et al., 2001).**

The ATN is in close anatomic relation to the condylar process, the TMJ, the superficial temporal artery (STA) and the LPt. ATN compression by hypertrophied LPt may result in neuralgia or paresthesia of TMJ, exernal acoustic meatus and facial muscles. Further it may result in functional impairment of salivation ipsilaterally. In addition, the altered position of the ATN and its extensive or multiple loops may render the ATN more liable to entrapment neuropathy. Temple headaches occur frequently due to entrapment of ATN, which sometimes is throbbing in nature, due to its proximity to STA **(Soni et al., 2009). Johannson et al. (1990)** revealed the existence of topographical prerequisites for mechanical influence upon the MN branches passing in the TMJ region. In joints, with a displaced disc, the ATN trunk was almost in contact with the medial aspect of the condyle instead of exhibiting its normal sheltered course at the level of the condylar neck, thus exposing the nerve possible mechanical irritation during anteromedial condylar movements.

The Inferior alveolar Nerve (IAN) normally descends medial to the LPt. At its lower border, the nerve passes between the SML and the mandibular ramus, and then enters the mandibular canal through the mandibular foramen. In the mandibular canal it runs downwards and forwards, generally below the apices of the teeth until below the first and second premolars, where it divides into the terminal incisive and mental branches **(Khan et al., 2009).** Because the IAN is a mixed nerve, it is suggested that during development, the sensory and motor fibres are guided separately, and take different migration pathways. When the motor component of the nerve leaves for its final destination, the sensory fibres reunite **(Krmpotic-Nemanic et al., 1999).** It was also found that the IAN and the LN may pass close to the medial part of the condyle. In joints with this nerve topography, a medially displaced disc could interfere mechanically with these nerves. These findings could explain the sharp, shooting pain felt locally in the joint with jaw movements and the pain and other sensations projecting to the terminal area of distribution of the nerve branches near the TMJ such as the ear, temple, cheek, tongue, and teeth **(Johansson et al., 1990).**

The Mylohyoid Nerve branches from the IAN as the latter descends between the SML and the mandibular ramus. The mylohyoid nerve (motor nerve) passes forward in a groove to reach the mylohyoid muscle and the anterior belly of the digastric muscle. **Loughner et al. (1990)** found an unusual entrapment of the mylohyoid nerve in the LPt in one cadaver. Nerve compression may cause a poorly localized deep pain from the muscles it innervates. Chronic compression of the nerve results in muscular paresis. Nerve entrapment bilaterally may provoke swallowing difficulties.

The Lingual Nerve (LN) is the smallest sensory branch of the posterior trunk of the MN. Below the FO, it is united closely with the IAN. Separating from the IAN, usually 5-10mm below the cranial base, it begins its course from the ITF near the otic ganglion **(Kim et al., 2004).** Data on LN topography in the ITF remain incomplete **(Trost et al., 2009).** LN runs between the tensor veli palatine and the LPt where it is joined by the chorda tympani (CT) (branch of the FN). The CT carrying taste fibres for the anterior two-thirds of the tongue and parasympathetic fibres to the submandibular and sublingual salivary glands **(Zur et al., 2004).** The LN emerging from the cover of the LPt, proceeds down and forwards lying on the surface of the MPt and moves progressively closer to the medial surface of the mandibular ramus until it is intimately related to the bone a few millimetres below and behind the junction of the vertical and horizontal mandible rami. Here, it lies anterior to, and slightly deeper than, the IAN. It then passes below the mandibular attachment of the superior pharyngeal constrictor and pterygomandibular raphe, closely applied to the periosteum of the medial surface of the mandible, until it lies opposite the posterior root of the 3rd molar tooth, where it is covered only by the gingival mucoperiosteum. At the level of the upper end of the mylohyoid line, the nerve turns in a sharp curve anteriorly to continue horizontally on the superior surface of the mylohyoid muscle into the oral cavity. The LN is, at this point in close relation with to the upper pole of the submandibular gland. Farther anteriorly, the LN lies close to the posterior part of the sublingual gland and then turns medially spiraling under the submandibular duct and divides into a variable number of branches, entering the substance of the tongue. The nerve lays first on styloglossus and then on the lateral surface of the hyoglossus and genioglossus, before dividing into terminal branches which supply the overlying lingual mucosa **(Peuker et al., 2001; Zur et al.,2004).** In addition to receiving the CT and a branch from the IAN, the LN is connected to the submandibular ganglion by two or three branches and at the anterior margin of the hyoglossus, it forms connecting loops with hypoglossal nerve twigs **(Gray's 1995).** The LN supplies general sensation to the mucosa, the floor of the mouth, the lingual gingiva and the mucosa of the anterior two thirds (presulcal part) of the tongue, being slightly overlapped posteriorly by lingual fibers of the glossopharyngeal nerve **(Rusu et al., 2008).** The nerve transfers neural sensory fibres for general sensitivity (pressure, temperature, pain, touch) and gustatory fibers for taste sensation to the anterior part of the tongue through the CT. The CT also carries preganglionic parasympathetic fibers providing secretomotor innervation to the submandibular, sublingual and minor salivary glands of the oral cavity **(Trost et al., 2009).** The medial and lateral branches bear anastomotic connections with the hypoglossal nerve in the tongue body. Knowledge of the precise anatomical distribution of the LN may aid the surgeon to ensure a safe and effective procedure **(Zur et al., 2009).** The LN can sometimes be entrapped, either through an ossified pterygospinous ligament, based on the outer part of the cranial base, or through an extremely wide lateral lamina of the pterygoid process of the sphenoid bone, or through the medial fibres of the lower belly of the LPt, or between the anterior margin of the pterygoid muscle and the mandibular lingual border or after its penetration in the MPt **(Loughner et al., 1990; Peuker et al., 2001; Von Ludinghausen et al., 2006) (Figures 3,4).** LN compression could lead to a weakening of taste transmission from the taste buds on the anterior two thirds of the tongue unilaterally **(Loughner et al., 1990; Kim et al., 2004).**

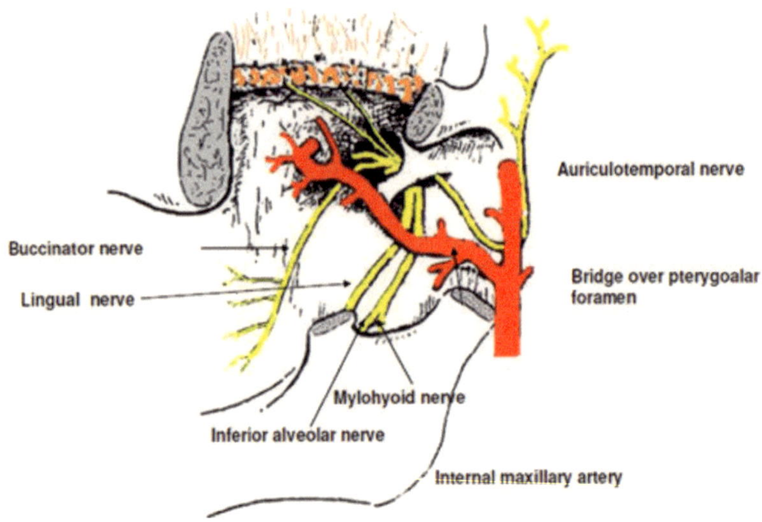

Fig. 3. The existence of pterygoalar foramen as a site of lingual nerve entrapment

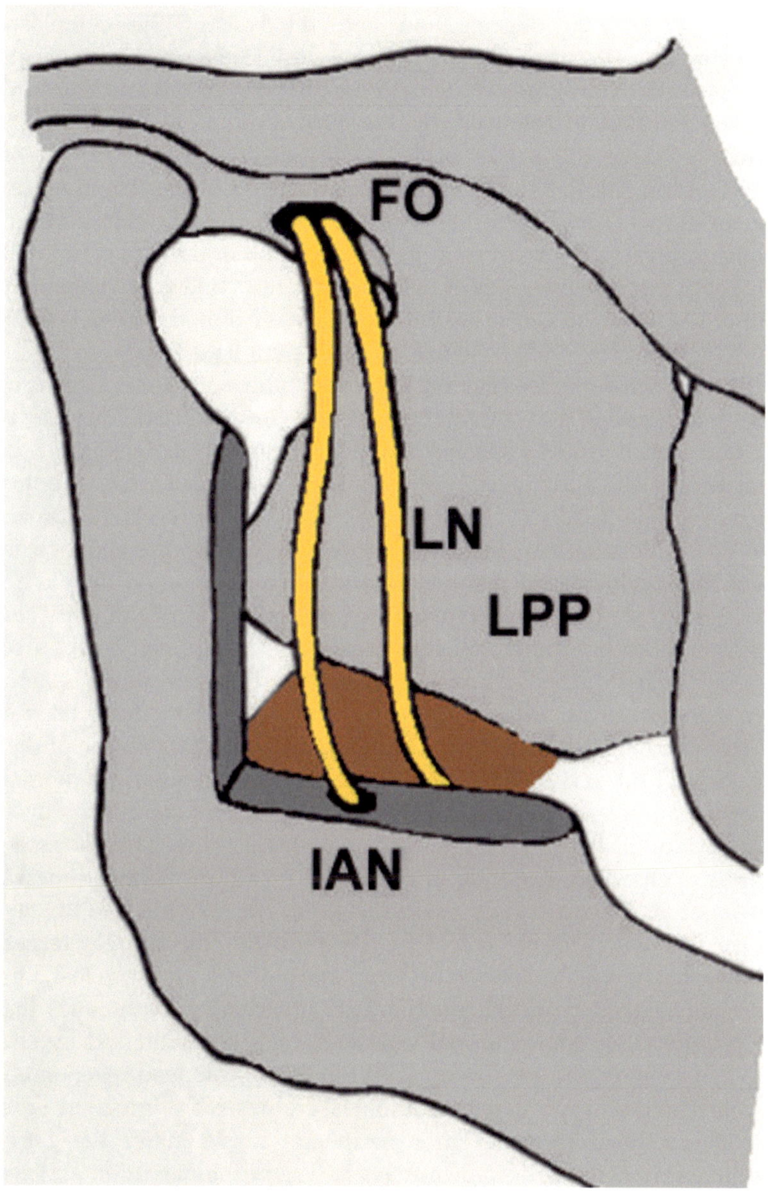

Fig. 4. A right ITF with a wide and large lateral pterygoid lamina

5. Reaction of neurons to injury

Reaction of neurons to physical trauma has been studied most extensively in motor neurons with peripheral axons, and centrally where their axons form well-defined tracts. When an axon is crushed or severed, changes occur on both sides of the lesion **(Nauta et al., 1974; Johnson et al., 2005).** Distally the axon initially swells and subsequently breaks up into a series of membrane-bound spheres. This process begins near the point of damage and progresses distally. These anterograde changes which also involve the axon terminal continue to total degeneration and removal of the cytoplasmic debris. Proximally, a similar series of changes may occur close to the point of injury, followed by a number of sequential, retrograde changes in the cell body **(Boyd and Gordon, 2003).** The process of degeneration is followed by the formation of new protein synthesizing organelles that produce distinctive proteins, destined for the regrowth of the axon **(Fenrich and Gordon, 2004).** Where regrowth of the axon is possible, the presence of an intact endoneurial sheath near to and beyond the region of injury is important if the axon is to reestablish satisfactory contact with its previous end organ or a closely adjacent one. The myelin sheath distal to the point of injury degenerates and is accompanied by mitotic proliferation of the Schwann cells, which fill the space inside the basal lamina of the old endoneurial tube **(Quarles, 2002).** Where a gap is present between the severed ends of the nerve, proliferating Schwann cells emerge from the stumps and form a series of nucleated cellular cords which bridge the interval **(Fenrich and Gordon,2004).** This may persist for a long time even in the absence of satisfactory nerve regeneration. Successful sprouts enter the proximal end of the endoneurial tube and grow distally in close contact with the surfaces of the Schwann cells it contains. This involves a process of contact guidance between the tip of the axon and the Schwann cell surfaces in the endoneurial tube and when present those which form Bungners bands. When the axon tip has reached and successfully reinnervated an end organ, the surrounding Schwann cells commence to synthesize myelin sheaths. Before full functional regeneration can occur, a considerable period of growth of both axonal diameter and myelin sheath thickness is necessary. This occurs when a high number of effective peripheral connections have been established. Regeneration of central axons does not normally occur, perhaps because of the absence of definite endoneurial tubes **(Fenrich and Gordon, 2004).** In general, when an axon is cut, Wallerian degeneration leads to axon degeneration and loss of conduction by 4 days. As a result of interruption of the post-ganglionic sympathetic efferent fibers, vaso- and sudo-motor paralysis is observed, resulting in red and dry skin in the area innervated by the nerve **(Johnson et al., 2005).** Various progressive changes take place in the target organs, skin blood vessels and sensory receptors. Peripherally, the muscle target losses its function, and centrally, motor neurons undergo atrophy and are often lost. One to 3 days after an axon is cut, the tips of the proximal stump forms growth cones that send out exploratory pseudopodia. Motor axonal regeneration is compromised by chronic distal nerve stump denervation, induced by delayed repair or prolonged regeneration distance, suggesting that the pathway for regeneration is progressively impaired with time and distance. Poor functional recovery after peripheral nerve injury has been generally attributed to inability of deneravated muscles to accept reinnervation and recover from denervation atrophy. On the other hand, deterioration of the environment produced by Schwann cells may play a more vital role. For the most part, atrophic Schwann cells retain their capacity to remyelinate regenerated axons, although they may loose their capacity to support axonal regeneration when chronically denervated. The importance of axonal regeneration through Schwann cell tubes surrounded by a basal lamina in the distal stump explains, in part, the different degrees of regeneration that are seen after crush injuries compared to transection. Although axons may be severed in crush injury, the Schwann cells, basal lamina and perineurium maintain continuity and, thus, facilitate regeneration. Considerable debate remains concerning the extent of axonal damage following chronic compression of axons **(Johnson et al., 2005).**

6. Mechanisms of entrapment neuropathies

Compression neuropathies are highly prevalent, debilitating conditions with variable functional recovery following surgical decompression. **Chronic nerve compression** induces concurrent Schwann cell proliferation and apoptosis in the early stages, without morphological and electrophysiological evidence of axonal damage. Proliferating Schwann cells down regulate myelin proteins, leading to local demyelination and remyelination in the region of injury. Axonal sprouting is related to the down regulation of myelin proteins, such as myelin-associated glycoprotein. This is contrast to acute crush or transection injuries, which are characterized by axonal injury followed by Wallerian degeneration **(Pham and Gupta, 2009).**

The posterior trunk of the MN might be entrapped occasionally from ligament's ossification between the lateral pterygoid process and the sphenoid spine near the FO **(Isberg et al., 1987; Loughner et al., 1990; Kapur et al., 2000).**

Although specific information regarding the clinical significance of ossified ligaments near the FO is limited, ossified ligaments appear to be very important from a practical clinical standpoint in relation to the different methods of block anesthesia of the MN **(Lepp and Sandner, 1968).** Additionally, these occasional structures may be important by producing various neurological disturbances **(Shaw, 1993). Krmpotic-Nemanic et al. (2001)** noted that a pterygospinous foramen replacing the FO could provoke trigeminal neuralgia **(Figure 5).**

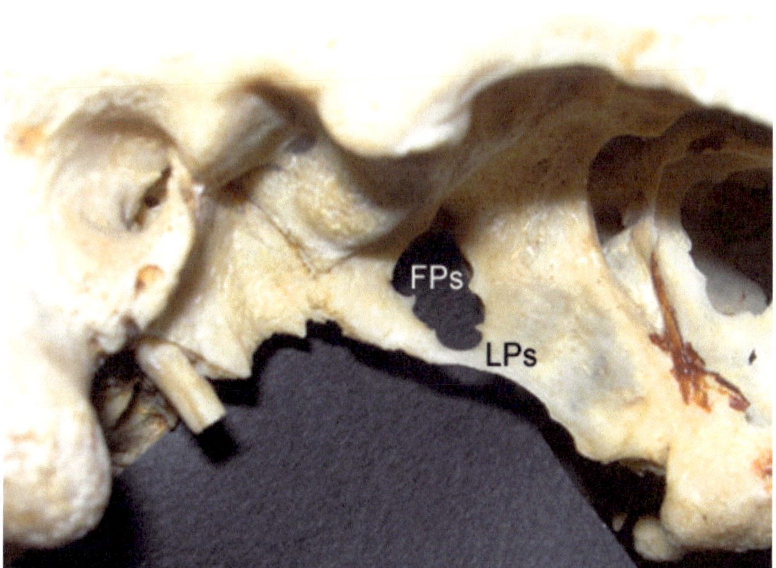

Fig. 5. Complete pterygospinous osseous bar and the enlarged pterygospinous foramen on the left side of a Greek dry skull

7. The injury of the lingual nerve (LN)

Injury to peripheral branches of the (TN) is a known sequelae of oral and maxillofacial surgical procedures. The two prime mechanisms of LN injury included crushing and transection. Although crush injuries are considered less severe than transection injuries, the axon distal to the injury site in both cases degenerates **(Sunderland, 1951).** However, unlike transection injuries, the connective tissue elements remain in continuity after crushing, which provides guidance for axonal sprouts from the regenerating central stump **(Sunderland, 1951; Johnson et al., 2005).** Injury to the LN is associated with changes in the epithelium of the tongue, particularly in the differentiation of the papillae and taste buds. Structural studies around the site of the injury show an apparent increase in the number of fascicles distal the crush site, suggesting considerable damage to the perineurium **(Holland et al., 1996).** The number of nonmyelinated axons distal to site of injury is double after crush injuries compared to control counts. This suggests that axonal sprouting persists for at least 12 weeks, with a rapid restoration of near-normal fibers for good functional recovery **(Holland et al., 1996).** Centrally, the principle change proximal to the nerve crush site is a loss of small-diameter myelinated axons from the chorda tympani. In addition, there is also an increase in the number of non-myelinated axons proximal to the crush site, indicative of continued sprouting following degeneration.

8. The entrapment of the lingual nerve (LN)

LN compression causes numbness, hypoesthesia, dysaesthesia, paraesthesia, or even anesthesia in all innervated regions. The patient may also present with dysgeusia, difficulty in chewing and loss of gustatory function on the side of the compression. Numbness of one lateral half or of the tip of the tongue can affect speech articulation of the frontal lingual consonants **(Isberg et al., 1987; Antonopoulou et al., 2008).** The LN can be entrapped, either through an ossified pterygospinous or pterygoalar ligament, based on the outer part of the cranial base, or through an extremely wide lateral lamina of the pterygoid process of the sphenoid bone, or through the medial fibers of the lower belly of the LPt **(Sunderland, 1991) (Figures 4, 6,7,8).** Recently, it is believed that, some cases of TMJ syndrome or myofascial pain syndrome could be a result of nerve entrapment in the ITF **(Kopell and Thompson, 1976; Von Ludinghausen et al., 2006).** A usual position of LN compression is the ITF contains the muscles of mastication, the pterygoid venous plexus, the MA and the ramification of the MN. The presence of a partially or completely ossified pterygospinous or pterygoalar ligament can obstruct the passage of a needle into the FO and disable the anesthesia of the trigeminal ganglion or the MN for relief of trigeminal neuralgia **(Lepp and Sandner, 1968; Skrzat et al., 2005) (Figures 5,6,7,8).** The presence of ossified LPs may compress the surrounding neurovascular structures causing lingual numbness and pain associated with speech impairment **(Peuker et al., 2001; Das and Paul, 2007).** Considering the close relationship of the CT, it may also be compressed by the anomalous bone bar and thus, result in abnormal taste sensation in the anterior two thirds of the tongue. The lateral lamina of the pterygoid process and the median pterygoid muscle forms the medial wall of the ITF. Elongation of the lateral lamina could result in weakening of the MPt and paresthesia of the buccal region **(Skrzat et al., 2006).** In cases of extremely large lateral laminae, the LN and IAN in the ITF are forced to take a longer more curved course, to follow the shape of the enlarged lamina. As a result, during contraction of the pterygoid muscles, both nerves can be compressed **(Figure 4).** The lateral pterygoid plate is an important landmark for mandibular anesthesia and a wide lateral pterygoid plate may confuse anesthetists or surgeons exploring the para- and retro-pharyngeal space **(Kapur et al., 2000; Das and Paul, 2007).**

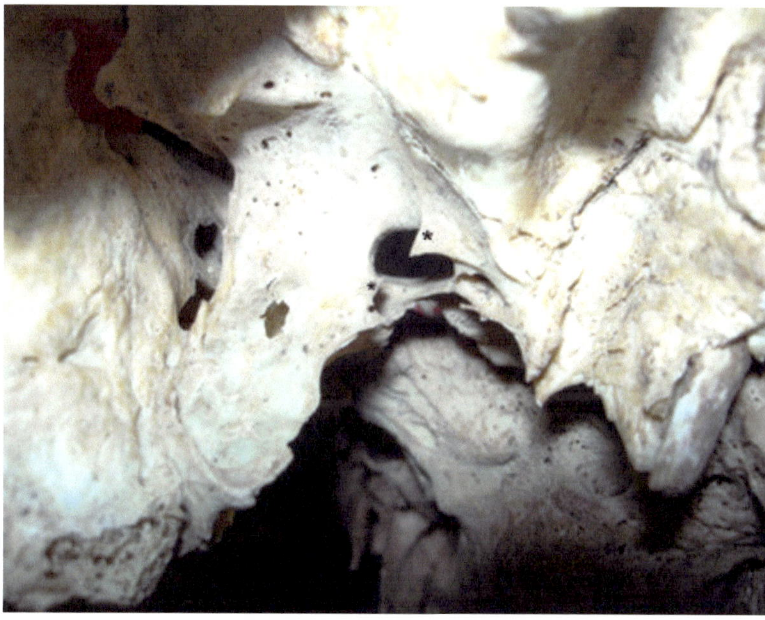

Fig. 6. Incomplete pterygospinous foramen on the left side of a Greek dry skull

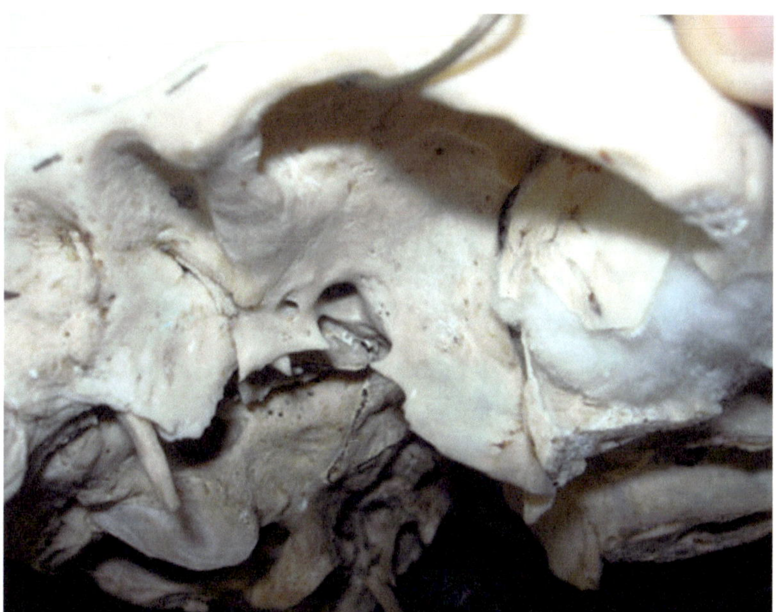

Fig. 7. Incomplete pterygoalar bar on the right side of a Greek dry skull

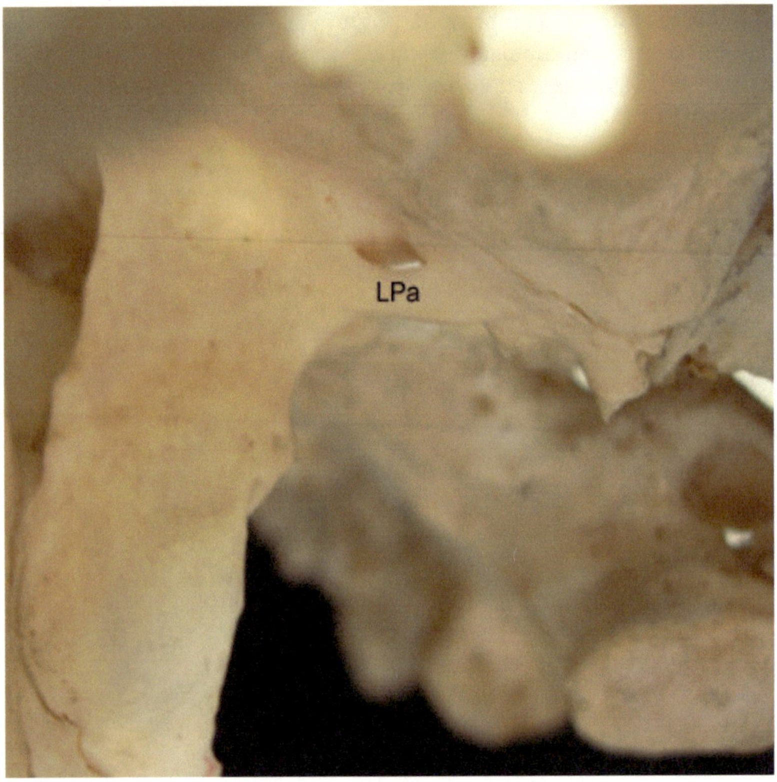

Fig. 8. Complete pterygoalar bar and a pterygoalar foramen on the left side of a Greek dry skull

LN entrapment can potentially occur between the median pterygoid bundles, or in the inferior head of the lateral pterygoid muscle, indicating that LPt spasm could cause LN compression and result in tongue numbness, anesthesia, or paresthesia at the tip of the tongue and speech articulation problems.

9. The entrapment of the remaining branches of the MN posterior trunk

An entrapped auriculotemporal nerve (ATN) in the lateral pterygoid muscle (LPt) could be the etiology behind a painful neuropathy in a distal ATN branch supplying sensory innervation to a deranged TMJ **(Akita et al., 2001).** The ATN is in close anatomic relation to the condylar process, the TMJ, the superficial temporal artery and the LPt. ATN compression by the hypertrophied LPt may result in neuralgia or paresthesia of TMJ, external acoustic meatus and facial muscles. Further it may result in functional impairment of salivation ipsilaterally. In addition, the altered position of the ATN and its extensive or multiple loops may render the ATN more liable to entrapment neuropathy. Temple headaches occur frequently due to entrapment of ATN, which sometimes is throbbing in nature, due to its proximity to superficial temporal artery **(Soni et al., 2009).** In joints, with a displaced disc, the ATN trunk can be almost in contact with the medial aspect of the condyle **(Johansson et al., 1990).** Thus, instead of exhibiting its normal sheltered course at the level of the condylar neck, the nerve is exposed to possible mechanical irritation during anteromedial condylar movements. Topographically, the **IAN** may pass close to the medial part of the condyle. As such, a medially displaced disc could interfere mechanically with this nerve. This could explain the sharp, shooting pain felt locally in the joint with jaw movements as well as the pain and other sensations projecting to the terminal area of distribution of the nerve branches near the TMJ, such as the ear, temple, cheek, tongue, and teeth **(Johansson et al., 1990).**

An unusual **entrapment of the mylohyoid nerve** in the LPt may cause a poorly localized deep pain from the muscles it innervates. Chronic compression of the nerve results in muscular paresis. This symptom would be subclinical unless the nerve entrapment is bilateral; then swallowing difficulties may ensue **(Loughner et al., 1990).**

10. Conclusions

Entrapment neuropathies are specific forms of compressive neuropathies occurring when nerves are confined to narrow anatomic passageways including soft and/or hard tissues making them susceptible to constricting pressures. Chronic nerve compression alters the normal anatomical and functional integrity of the nerve. Dentists and oral maxillofacial surgeons should be very suspicious of possible signs of neurovascular compression in the region of the ITF.

11. References

Akita K, Shimokawa T, Sato T. 2000. Positional relationships between the masticatory muscles and their innervating nerves with special reference to the lateral pterygoid and the midmedial and discotemporal muscle bundles of temporalis. J Anat 197: 291-302.

Akita K, Shimokawa T, Sato T. 2001. Aberrant muscle between the Temporalis and the Lateral Pterygoid Muscles: M. pterygoideus proprius (Henle). Clin Anat 14: 288-291.

Anil A, Peker T, Turgut HB, Gulekon IN, Liman F. 2003. Variations in the anatomy of the inferior alveolar nerve. British Journal of Oral and Maxillofacial Surgery 41: 236-239.

Antonopoulou M, Piagkou M, Anagnostopoulou S. 2008. An anatomical study of the pterygospinous and pterygoalar bars and foramina- their clinical relevance. Journal of Cranio-Maxillofacial Surgery 36: 104-108.

Boyd JG, Gordon T. 2003. Neurotrophic factors and their receptors in axonal regeneration and functional recovery after peripheral nerve injury. Mol Neurobiol 27:277–324.

Das S, Paul S. 2007. Ossified pterygospinous ligament and its clinical implications. Bratisl Lek Listy 108:141–143.

De Froe, Wagennar JH. 1935. Die Bedeutung des porus crotaphitico-buccinatorius and des Foramen pterygospinosum fur Neurologic and Rontgenologic

Fenrich K, Gordon T. 2004. Canadian Association of Neuroscience review: Axonal regeneration in the peripheral and central nervous systems—current issues and advances. Can J Neurol Sci 31:142–156.

Gray's Anatomy. 1995. Churchill Livingstone, New York, 28th edition, p. 380-381.

Holland GR, Robinson PP, Smith KG, Pehowich E. 1996. A quantitative morphological study of the recovery of cat lingual nerves after transection or crushing. J Anat 188:289–297.

Isberg AM, Isacsson G, Williams WN, Loughner BA. 1987. Lingual numbness and speech articulation deviation associated with temporomandibular joint disk displacement. Oral Surg Oral Med Oral Pathol 64: 9-14.

Johansson AS, Isberg A, Isacsson G. 1990. A radiographic and histologic study of the topographic relations in the temporomandibular joint region: implications for a nerve entrapment mechanism. J Oral Maxillofac Surg 48: 953-961.

Johnson EO, Zoubos AB, Soucacos PN. 2005. Regeneration and repair of peripheral nerves. Injury 36 Suppl 4:S24–S29.

Kapur E, Dilberovic F, Redzepagic S, Berhamovic E. 2000. Variation in the lateral plate of the pterygoid process and the lateral subzygomatic approach to the mandibular nerve. Med Arh 54: 133-137.

Khan MM, Darwish HH, Zaher WA. 2009. Perforation of the inferior alveolar nerve by the maxillary artery: An anatomical study. British Journal of Oral and Maxillofacial Surgery (in Press)

Kim HJ, Kwak HH, Hu KS, Park HD, Kang HC, Jung HS, Koh KS. 2003. Topographic anatomy of the mandibular nerve branches distributed on the two heads of the lateral pterygoid. Int J. Oral Maxillofac. Surg 32: 408-413.

Kim SY, Hu KS, Chung IH, Lee EW, Kim HJ. 2004. Topographic anatomy of the lingual nerve and variations in communication pattern of the mandibular nerve branches. Surg Radiol Anat 26: 128-135.

Kopell HP, Thompson WAL. 1976. Peripheral Entrapment Neuropathies. Huntington, New York: Krieger Publishing Company. p 1–7.

Krmpotic - Nemanic J, Vinter J, Jalsovec D. 2001. Accessory oval foramen. Ann Anat 183: 293-295

Krmpotic-Nemanic J, Vinter I, Hat J, Jalsovec D. 1999. Mandibular neuralgia due to anatomical variations. Eur Arch Otorh 256: 205-208

Kwak HH, Ko SJ, Jung HS, Park HD, Chung IH, Kim HJ. 2003. Topographic anatomy of the deep temporal nerves, with references to the superior head of lateral pterygoid. Surg Radiol Anat 25: 393-399

Lang J. 1995. Skull base and related structures - Atlas of Clinical Anatomy. Stuttgart, Schattauer; p. 55-57, 300-311

Lang J, Hetterich A. 1983. Contribution on the postnatal development of the processus pterygoideus. Anat Anz 154: 1-31

Lepp FH, Sandner O. 1968. Anatomic-radiographic study of ossi.ed pterygospinous and 'innominate' ligaments. Oral Surg Oral Med Oral Pathol 26:244–260.

Loughner BA, Larkin LH, Mahan PE. 1990. Nerve entrapment in the lateral pterygoid muscle. Oral Surg Oral Med Oral Pathol 69:299–306.

Madhavi C, Issac B, Jacob TM. 2006. Variation of the middle deep temporal nerve: A case report. Eur J Anat 10: 157-160

Nauta HJ, Pritz MB, Lasek RJ. 1974. Afferents to the rat caudoputamen studied with horseradish peroxidase: An evaluation of retrograde neuroanatomical research methods. Brain Res 67:219- 238.

Nayak SR, Rai R, Krishnamurthy A, Prabhu LV, Ranade AV, Mansur DI, Kumar S. 2008. An unusual course and entrapment of the lingual nerve in the infratemporal fossa. Bratisl Lek Listy 109: 525-527

Nayak SR, Saralaya V, Prabhu LV, Pai MM, Vadgaonkar R, D' Costa S. 2007. Pterygospinous bar and foramina in Indian skulls: incidence and phylogenetic significance. Surg Radiol Anat 29: 5-7

Newton TH, Potts DG (1971) Radiology of the skull and brain. Vol.1. St Louis: I. Mosby, p. 307

Ozdogmus O, Saka E, Tulay C, Gurdal E, Uzun I, Cavdar S (2003) The anatomy of the carotico-clinoid foramen and its relation with the internal carotid artery. Surg Radiol Anat 25: 241-246

Patnaik VVG, Singla Rajan K, Bala Sanju (2001) Bilateral pterygoalar bar and porus crotaphitico-buccinatorius- a case report. J Anat. Soc. India 50: 161-162

Peker T, Karakose M, Anil A, Turgut H.B, Gulekon N (2002) The incidence of basal sphenoid bony bridges in dried crania and cadavers: Their anthropological and clinical relevance. Eur J Morphol 40: 171-80

Peuker ET, Fischer G, Filler TJ. 2001. Entrapment of the lingual nerve due to an ossified pterygospinous ligament. Clin Anat 14:282–284.

Pham K, Gupta R. 2009. Understanding the mechanisms of entrapment neuropathies. Review article. Neurosurg Focus 26:E7.

Piagkou M, Demesticha T, Piagkos G, Androutsos G, Skandalakis P. 2011. Mandibular nerve entrapment in the infratemporal fossa. Surg Radiol Anat 33: 291-299.

Piagkou M, Demesticha T, Piagkos G, Androutsos G, Skandalakis P. 2010. Lingual nerve entrapment in muscular and osseous structures. IJOS 2 (4): 181-189.

Pinar Y, Arsu G, Aktan Ikiz za, Bilge O (2004) Pterygospinous and pterygoalar bridges. Sendrom 16; 66-69

Prades JM, Timishenko A, Merzougui N (2003) A cadaveric study of a combined trans-mandibular and trans-zygomatic approach to the infratemporal fossa. Surg Radiol Anat 25: 180-187

Quarles RH. 2002. Myelin sheaths: Glycoproteins involved in their formation, maintenance and degeneration. Cell Mol Life Sci 59:1851–1871.

Rusu MC, Nimigean V, Podoleanu L, Ivascu RV, Niculescu MC. 2008. Details of the intralingual topography and morphology of the lingual nerve. Int J Oral Maxillofac Surg 37:835–839.

Sakamoto Y, Akita K. 2004. Spatial relationships between masticatory muscles and their innervating nerves in man with special reference to the medial pterygoid muscle and its accessory muscle bundle. Surg Radiol Anat 26:122–127

Shaw JP. 1993. Pterygospinous and pterygoalar foramina: A Role in the etiology of Trigeminal Neuralgia? Clin Anat 6: 173-178

Shaw JP. 1993. Pterygospinous and pterygoalar foramina: A role in the etiology of trigeminal neuralgia? Clin Anat 6:173–178.

Shimokawa T, Akita K, Sato T, Ru F, Yi SQ, Tanaka S. 2004. Penetration of muscles by branches of the mandibular nerve: A possible cause of neuropathy. Clin Anat 17:2-5.

Shimokawa T, Akita K, Soma K, Sato T. 1998. Innervation analysis of the small muscle bundles attached to the temporalis: truly new muscles or merely derivatives of the temporalis? Surg Radiol Anat 20: 329-334

Skrzat J, Walocha J, Srodek R. 2005. An anatomical study of the pterygoalar bar and the pterygoalar foramen. Folia Morphol 64: 92-96

Skrzat J, Walocha J, Srodek R, Nizankowska A. 2006. An atypical position of the foramen ovale. Folia Morphol 65:396–399.

Skrzat J,Walocha J, Srodek R. 2005. An anatomical study of the pterygoalar bar and the pterygoalar foramen. Folia Morphol 64:92–96.

Soni S, Rath G, Suri R, Vollala VR (2009) Unusual organization of Auriculotemporal Nerve and Its Clinical Implications. Journal of Oral and Maxillofacial Surgery 67: 448-450

Sunderland S (1991) Nerve injuries and their repair: a critical appraisal. Churchill Livingstone, New York, p. 129–146

Sunderland S. 1951. A classification of peripheral nerve injuries producing loss of function. Brain 74:491–516.

Sutherland S (1978) Nerves and nerve injuries. New York: Churchill Livingstone, p. 343-350

Tebo HG (1968) The pterygospinous bar in panoramic roentgenography. Oral Surg Oral Med Oral Pathol 26: 654-657

Trost O, Kazemi A, Cheynel N, Benkhadra M, Soichot P, Malka G, Trouilloud P (2009) Spatial relatioships between linbgual nerve and mandibular ramus: original study method, clinical and educational applications. Surg Radiol Anat 31: 447-452

Tubbs RS, May WR Jr, Apaydin N, Shoja MM, Shokouhi G, Loukas M, Cohen-Gadol AA. 2009. Ossification of ligaments near the foramen ovale: An anatomic study with potential clinical significance regarding transcutaenous approaches to the skull base. Neurosurgery 65(6 Suppl):60–64.

Von Ludinghausen M, Kageyama I, Miura M, Al Khatib M (2006) Morphological pecularities on the deep infratemporal fossa in advanced age. Surg Radiol Anat 28: 284-292

Yoshimasu F, Kurland LT, Elveback LR (1972) Tic douloureux in Rochester, Minnesota, 1945-1969. Neurology, 22: 952-956

Zakrzewska JM (1990) Medical management of trigeminal neuralgia. Br Dent J 168: 399-401

Zur KB, Mu L, Sanders I. 2004. Distribution pattern of the human lingual nerve. Clin Anat 17:88–92.